POTTENGER'S CATS

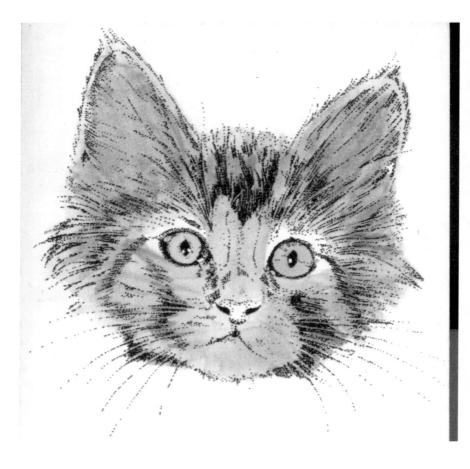

Cover from original 1983 edition. Illustration by Roxanne Pottenger.

POTTENGER'S CATS

A Study in Nutrition

By Francis M. Pottenger, Jr., M.D.

Edited by

Elaine Pottenger

with

Robert T. Pottenger, Jr., M.D.

Address:	7890 Broadway
	Lemon Grove, CA 91945
Phone:	(800) 366-3748
	(619) 462-7600
Fax:	(619) 433-3136

ISBN 13: 978-0-916764-06-7

Library of Congress Catalog Card Number: 83-80360

Manufactured in the United States of America

Note to Researchers:
Price-Pottenger makes available reprints (117) of the professional reports by
Francis Marion Pottenger, Jr., M.D., upon which this book was based. We are able
to make available reprints (178) of his father, Francis Marion Pottenger, Sr., M.D.'s
work as well. Many of these papers are available exclusively to members at
price-pottenger.org. The foundation has additional archival documents from their
research, including some X-rays.

Website: www.price-pottenger.org
Email: info@price-pottenger.org

Dedication

This book is dedicated to the cats and the memories of Francis M. Pottenger, Jr., M.D., Weston A. Price, D.D.S., William A. Albrecht, Ph.D., and all the pioneers in the fields of nutrition, agronomy, and animal husbandry. May today's scientists continue in the pursuit of the knowledge uncovered by these pioneers in the early twentieth century.

The greatest gift to this earth is the knowledge we leave behind for others. May we look at this scientific research not only for what it can do for the health of our animals, but also for what it can do for the health and happiness of all creatures great and small.

Sponsors

American Academy of Nutrition
  Golden Gate Chapter
Radford Bivans
Don & Jeanette Brancaccio
  A-1 Nutrition Store
Vincent L. Briggs
Cecyl Bruner
Ruby Price Chuck
Anne E. Clay
Jackie Cooper
Alsoph H. Corwin
Elias N. Costianes
David Crystal, D.D.S.
Maureen F. Curtis
William H. Fisher, D.D.S.
Willis & Jane Fletcher Foundation
Sanford C. Frumker, D.D.S.
Keith M. & Antha Newport Harnish
Dr. & Mrs. Joseph Harvey Harris
Helen Pottenger Hops
V. Earl & Julia O. Irons
Douglas W. Kerr, D.D.S.
Mr. & Mrs. Ted Knight
Mr. & Mrs. Ross Le Lansky
Ronald M. Lesko, D.O.
William C. Maul
Carlyle Miller, D.D.S.

L. R. Misner, Jr., D.D.S.
John A. Myers, M.D.
Dr. Marita H. Neiss
Carl and Cloey Niemack
R. W. Noble, M.D.
Robert Null, M.D.
Parents for Better Nutrition
  (Thelma Thompson)
Dr. Olympio Fassol Pinto
Louise S. Porter
In memory of Joseph Risser, M.D.
  – Risser Orthopedic Research, Inc.
Mrs. F. B. Rosevear
Michael B. Schachter
Audrey M. Schneider
John & Valerie Scudder
Allison C. Sedgwick
Harold N. Simpson
Quentin M. Stephen-Hassard, D.D.S.
Mr. & Mrs. Leland (Reba) Stone
Ted Sundahl
H. Grant and Jacquette S. Theis
Charles A. Walker
Westgate Health Foods, Inc.
Charles Zahn
Jeffrey S. Zavik

Price-Pottenger and the authors wish to acknowledge and thank Dr. Donald Kelley and Philip Kelley for contributing their time and equipment for the original typesetting of this book. Their generosity in the face of numerous difficulties was far more than the call of duty.

The second printing was facilitated through the generosity of John and Frieda Mattingly.

Acknowledgments

The purpose of this book is to unify the work of Francis M. Pottenger, Jr., M.D., and to help remove the confusion sometimes found in the lay literature as to the actual scope and results of his research.

We would like to acknowledge the extensive reprint library of Francis M. Pottenger, Jr., as made available to us through Price-Pottenger, to acknowledge the help and encouragement of Pat Connolly, Curator of the Foundation, and the help of her dedicated staff, and to acknowledge the assistance of a former Foundation staff member, Betty Jean King.

We would like to acknowledge the members of the Board of Directors of Price-Pottenger who have provided continuing support from the start to the finish of this book and to extend special appreciation to those whose generous donations made the publication of this book possible.

Finally, we would like to recognize the assistance of Mrs. Dorothy Pottenger and Mrs. Helen Pottenger Hops who read the manuscript in progress and offered valuable information and insight from their personal knowledge of the work of Francis M. Pottenger, Jr.

While all the facts herein are carefully researched and verified, any errors of presentation or interpretation are those of the editors.

PRICE ℞ POTTENGER

Changing lives through **health and nutrition**

Our Mission:

To educate people on the remarkable benefits of a natural plant- and animal-based diet and inspire individuals to live a healthy lifestyle.

Our History:

Price-Pottenger is a leading resource for practical and current information on traditional diets, food preparation, organic foods, environmental influences, various health conditions, and more.

Founded in 1952 as the Santa Barbara Medical Research Foundation, we later became the Weston A. Price Memorial Foundation in 1966.

Our name was changed to The Price-Pottenger Nutrition Foundation in 1973 to honor the invaluable contributions made by both Weston A. Price, DDS, and Francis M. Pottenger, Jr., MD. Price-Pottenger is the repository for their research and that of others who augment their philosophies. The foundation continues to publish Dr. Price's *Nutrition and Physical Degeneration*; *Dental Infections, Oral and Systemic*; and *Dental Infections & the Degenerative Diseases*; as well as Dr. Pottenger's classic experiment, Pottenger's Cats: A Study in Nutrition.

We simplified our name to Price-Pottenger in 2016 to reflect the wide appeal the foundation has achieved.

We are a nonprofit, 501(c)(3) public education corporation supported by subscriptions, donations, and sales of educational materials.

Members have online access to video courses, guidance, tips, articles, and classes on nutrition and a wide variety of other topics to make it easier for them to live a healthier lifestyle.

Professional members also receive a free listing on our website to help them connect with clients.

Preface

Conceptual visualization in scientific research is rare. Francis M. Pottenger, Jr., had such vision. Dedicated to the cause of preventing chronic illness, he made significant contributions to the understanding of the role nutrition plays in maintaining good health.

Francis conceived long-term studies concerning the effect of the supply of nutrients on the growth and development of musculoskeletal structures using felines for his experimental animals. With the aid of biological and Roentgen studies, he showed how deficiencies in nutrition lead to deficiencies in bone maturation by affecting the adrenal and thyroid glands.

More than any other single individual, Francis was responsible for opening what resembled a Pandora's Box of research concerning nutrition and its effects on body function and growth. His work preceded Albright's notable publications on calcium and the Mayo Clinic publications on cortisone.

As the Pottenger research progressed, the significance of his studies broadened. It soon became evident that a correlation could be made between the quality of nutrition in childhood and the ability of the adult to handle stress. A similar correlation was later made by Levine in his adrenal development and stress studies at Stanford.

The importance of the quality of milk in supplying adequate calcium to bone development was also demonstrated in the Pottenger feline studies. It is a pleasure to note that recent literature has been tending to recognize this.

Harvey E. Billig, Jr., M.D., F.I.C.S., F.A.C.S.M.

Table of Contents

Cereals and Breadstuffs
Beverages
Meats
Vegetables
Fruits
Desserts
Recipe A — Gelatin
Recipe B — Liver
Recipe C — Brains
Recipe D — Fresh Ground Beef
Recipe E — Variety Meats Other than Liver and Brains
Recipe F — Soup
Recipe G — Sprouting Beans and Grains

List of Tables

Glossary

Acini	Pl. of acinus—one of the small sacs in a gland lining with secreting cells
Agnathia	A developmental anomaly characterized by total or virtual absence of lower jaw
Albumin	A protein found in every animal and in many vegetable tissues
Albuminoid	Resembling albumin
Alopecia	Baldness, deficiency of hair, natural or abnormal
Alveolar	Of, relating to, or constituting the part of the jaws where the teeth arise, ridge containing sockets of teeth
Amnion	The thin, transparent, tough silver membrane lining of the placenta that produces, at the earliest period of fetation, the amniotic fluid
Amniotic sac	Membrane containing amniotic fluid
Anemia	A condition in which the blood is deficient either in quantity or quality
Apices	Pl. of apex—the top or pointed extremity
Atelectasis	Incomplete expansion of lungs at birth
Atheroma	Fatty degeneration of the inner coat of arteries
Atrophy	A defect or failure of nutrition manifested as a wasting away or diminution in the size of a cell, tissue, organ, or part
Bronchitis	Acute or chronic inflammation of the bronchial tubes
Calcaneus	Heel bone
Carpal	Of or pertaining to the wrist
Colloid	Glutinous or resembling glue; a state of matter in which the matter is dispersed in or distributed throughout some medium called the dispersion medium
Cortex	Outer layer of an organ
Cuboid	Resembling a cube
Cuneiform	Triangular
Deciduous	Not permanent
Electrolytic	Pertaining to electrolysis, the passage of a stream of electricity through a solution that conducts electricity by means of its ion
Empyema	Accumulation of pus in a cavity of body, especially the chest
Enteral	Within, or by way of, the intestine
Epiphysis	A piece of bone separated from a long bone in early life by cartilage, but later becoming a part of the larger bone. It is at this cartilaginous joint that growth in length of the bone occurs.
Excreta	Manure
Gingivitis	Inflammation of the gum
Globulins	A class of proteins characterized by being insoluble in water

Hamate	Unciform (hook-shaped) bone at the ulnar edge of the carpus
Hydrophilic	Readily absorbing moisture
Hyperemia	Excess of blood in any part of the body
Hyperplasia	The abnormal increase in the number of normal cells in normal arrangement in tissues
Hypothyroidism	Deficient activity of the thyroid gland
Immunology	Study of immunity
Lingual	Pertaining to the tongue
Lunate	Semilunar bone
Malar	Pertaining to the cheek or cheek bone
Mandible	The horseshoe-shaped bone forming the lower jaw
Masseter	Muscle that raises the mandible and closes the jaw
Maxilla	Upper jaw
Metacarpal	The part of the hand between the wrist and fingers
Nares	The openings into the nasal cavity
Navicular	Scaphoid or boat-shaped
Nucha	The back, nape, or scruff of the neck
Osseous	Pertaining to bone
Osteogenesis imperfecta	An inherited condition in which bones are abnormally brittle and subject to fractures
Osteoporosis	Abnormal porousness of bone by enlargement of its canals or by the formation of abnormal spaces
Pathology	Study of essential nature of disease, the structural and functional changes in tissues
Physiology	Study of the functions of the living organism and its parts
Pneumonitis	Localized acute inflammation of the lungs without toxemia
Polymerize	The process of forming a compound, usually of higher molecular weight, by the combination of simpler molecules
Pterygoid	Shaped like a wing
Pyorrhea	Discharge of pus
Ramus	A branch, as of an artery, bone, nerve, or vein
Reproductive Efficiency	Ability of a female to become pregnant, deliver, and nurse viable offspring. Fertility of a male.
Signs	Physical findings
Spermatozoa	Male germ cells
Spermatogenesis	Process of formation of spermatozoa
Suture	Line of union in an immovable articulation, as between bones of the skull
Symptoms	Complaints
Trabeculation	Internal structural mesh of bones
Viscera	Pl. of viscus—any large interior organ in any one of three great body cavities, especially the abdomen
Zygoma	Arch formed by zygomatic process of the temporal bone and by the malar bone

Introduction

Between the years of 1932 and 1942, Dr. Francis Marion Pottenger, Jr., conducted a feeding experiment to determine the effects of heat-processed food on cats. His ten-year cat study was prompted by the high rate of mortality he was experiencing among his laboratory cats undergoing adrenalectomies during his efforts to standardize the hormone content of an adrenal extract he was making. Because there were no existent chemical procedures for standardizing biological extracts, manufacturers of such extracts necessarily had to use animals to determine their potency. Since cats die without their adrenal glands, the dose of extract required to support their lives calibrated the level of the extract's potency.

In his effort to maximize the preoperative health of his laboratory animals, Francis fed them a diet of market-grade raw milk, cod liver oil, and scraps of *cooked meat* from the sanatorium. These scraps included liver, tripe, sweetbreads, brain, heart, and muscle. This diet was considered by the experts of the day to be rich in all the important nutritive substances, and the surgical technique used for the adrenalectomies was the most exacting known. Therefore, Francis was perplexed as to why his cats were poor operative risks. In seeking an explanation, he began noticing that the cats showed signs of deficiency. All showed a decrease in their reproductive capacity, and many of the kittens born in the laboratory had skeletal deformities and organ malfunctions.

As his neighbors in Monrovia kept donating an increasing number of cats to his laboratory, the demand for scraps of cooked meat exceeded his supply, so he placed an order at the local meat packing plant for scraps of *raw meat*, again including the viscera, muscle, and bone. These raw-meat scraps were fed to a segregated group of cats each day, and within a few months, this group appeared in better health than the animals being fed scraps of cooked meat. Their kittens appeared more vigorous, and most interestingly, their operative mortality decreased markedly.

The contrast in the apparent health of the cats fed raw meat and those fed cooked meat was so startling, it prompted Francis to undertake a controlled experiment. What he had observed by chance, he wanted to repeat by design. He wanted to find answers to such questions as: Why did the cats eating raw meat survive their operations more readily than those eating cooked meat? Why did the kittens of the cats fed raw meat appear more vigorous? Why did a diet based on scraps of cooked meat apparently fail to provide the necessary nutritional elements for good health? He felt the findings of a controlled feeding experiment might illumine new facts about optimal human nutrition.

The Cat Study of Francis Pottenger, Jr., is unique. There is no similar experiment in the medical literature. The pathological and chemical findings were supervised by Francis in consultation with Alvin G. Foord, M.D., professor of pathology at the University of Southern California and a pathologist at the Huntington Memorial Hospital in Pasadena. Accordingly, the studies met the most rigorous scientific standards of the day, and their protocol was observed consistently.

Since The Cat Study is unique, its findings are frequently quoted and misquoted in order to justify the ideas of others. For example, one author of a popular-selling book states that 200 cats died of arthritis; this indeed did not happen. Another author states that the cats were fed sprouts and survived in full health for four continuous generations. Again, no such experiment took place, and yet this misinformation has been traced over a dozen or more different articles and books.

A frequent criticism of The Pottenger Cat Study is that it was not properly controlled. Here it is necessary to ask, "By what standards?" Every one of the studies followed strictly defined protocol. All variables in the stock of the animals were reported and explained. Because some of the test procedures may seem crude forty years later, this in no way invalidates the facts that the procedures were meticulously controlled and that the results of the experiments were reported as observed.

Another criticism is that the cats were kept in an artificial environment unrelated to real living conditions. Such a criticism overlooks the experimental necessity of maintaining a controlled environment to provide valid findings. It also overlooks the evidence that, given specific living conditions, specific changes *repeatedly* occurred in the health of the cats under observation.

Another frequent criticism is that the experimental work done on cat nutrition has no appropriate application to human nutrition. Francis Pottenger, Jr., never stated that a one-to-one comparison could be made between his findings in cat nutrition and his findings in human nutrition. He did say: "While no attempt will be made to correlate the changes in the animals studied with malformations found in humans, the similarity is so obvious that parallel pictures will suggest themselves."

All too often, self-appointed authorities will state categorically that they do not believe others' observations and so seek to close the door on any further inquiry into these observations. They declare, "Because I do not believe the facts as presented, they are not so." Far better for science if responsible individuals maintain an attitude of open inquiry and test the observations of others before forming rigid opinions. In the case of The Cat Study, human welfare might well be served if concerned researchers made every effort to discover if valid correlations can be made between cat nutrition and human nutrition. It must be remembered that cats and humans both are mammalian biological systems.

It would be of great value to the field of nutrition to repeat The Cat Study within the parameters of present-day technology and with the use of present-day antibiotics. Most of the cats on deficient diets died from infections of the kidneys, lungs, and bones. If these infections were eliminated as a cause of death by antibiotics, it would allow the cats to reveal their ultimate degenerative fates. As an extension to this experiment, it would be of interest to study the effects of vitamin and mineral supplementation in the diet of animals fed cooked food.*

It is our effort in this monograph to present the observations made by Francis M. Pottenger, Jr., on the effects of deficient and optimum nutrition in cats and human beings as recorded in his articles and clinical records written between the years of 1932 and 1956. Nothing has been added or subtracted from his findings, and for the most part, the words describing his work are his own. Though some of the scientific *interpretations* have not withstood the test of time, the *observations* are valid. A careful and selective interpretation by an inquiring mind will readily differentiate the two.

---

*Price-Pottenger is interested in research repeating The Cat Study and any related experiments.

The text of Part I, Part II, and Part III is taken from the published articles of Francis M. Pottenger, Jr., listed in italics at the beginning of each chapter. The articles are available for purchase from Price-Pottenger. Their text has been edited and integrated for the purposes of this presentation; however, the writing is largely in its original form.

Part One

Cat Nutrition

Chapter One

THE POTTENGER CAT STUDY

"The Effect of Heat-Processed Foods and Metabolized Vitamin D Milk on Dento-facial Structures of Experimental Animals," "The Influence of Heat Labile Factors on Nutrition in Oral Development and Health."

The cats in The Pottenger Cat Study were kept in large outdoor pens. The pens were built near a stand of eucalyptus trees on a side of a hill overlooking the San Gabriel Valley. Each pen had an open-air enclosure 12 feet long, 6 feet wide, and 7 feet high, which was screened by chicken-wire so the cats had adequate exposure to the sun. A trench 18 inches deep was dug in each enclosure and filled with freshly washed sand from a common sand pile. A roofed area approximately 4-feet deep with a wooden floor and bedding extended from the back of each pen to provide shelter for the animals during inclement weather. A caretaker removed bones and uneaten food daily, and cleaned and refilled the water containers. Periodically, he removed the cats' buried excreta from the sand for composting in piles marked according to the cats' diet.

All animals were subject to the same routine procedures. Each cat had its own clinical chart, and notes were kept throughout its life. All cats were weighed, numbered, and described. In the cases of donated animals, all possible information was obtained from their donors regarding their histories of development, the types of food they had received from birth, and their general condition of health. The kittens born of experimental animals were carefully described, and their birth dates and lineage were recorded along with any delivery problems the mother cat experienced. Kittens born dead were subject to immediate autopsy and examined for any abnormalities or birth defects, either by the naked eye or through a microscope. Such postmortem examinations accompanied the death of all cats.

5

X-ray studies were made of some of the cats in order to study the effects of the various experimental diets on their skeletal development. Moreover, calcium and phosphorus determinations were made during the postmortems of most of the experimental animals. These determinations were confined basically to the size and weight of the femurs and the percentage of calcium and phosphorus in them.

At the end of ten years, 600 out of 900 cats studied had complete, recorded health histories. The majority of these records are in the archives of Price-Pottenger.

DEFINITIONS

As The Cat Study includes several generations of cats, it is necessary to understand how the different generations are classified before discussing the actual feeding experiments. In classifying the experimental animals, the word *diet* describes the actual food intake of the individual cat. An *optimum diet* refers to a diet of raw food, including raw meat, raw milk, and cod liver oil. A *deficient diet* refers to a diet that includes one or more cooked foods plus cod liver oil. Cod liver oil is routinely included in all experimental diets as a rich supplemental source of vitamin A.

According to the diet variables of raw or cooked foods, the cats are grouped in three general health classifications: (1) normal, (2) deficient, and (3) regenerating.

Normal Cats

Normal cats are born of healthy parents and are maintained on an optimum diet of raw food and cod liver oil. They are the control cats used for comparison with the deficient and regenerating cats. The breeding males used in the various experiments are always of this normal group and are of proven fertility so that experimental results primarily reflect the condition of the health of the mother cats.

Deficient Cats

First-Generation Deficient Cats: These cats are either mature cats donated to the study or mature cats born of experimental animals and raised on an optimum diet. When these adult cats are placed on deficient diets that include cooked food, they are called deficient cats of the first generation.

Second-Generation Deficient Cats: These cats are the kittens born to females of the first deficient generation eating a deficient diet for various lengths of time prior to and during gestation and lactation. At the end of nursing, these kittens are maintained on a deficient diet.

Third-Generation Deficient Cats: These cats are the kittens born of the second deficient generation and maintained on deficient diets all their lives.

Regenerating Cats

Regenerating Kittens of the First Order: When a female cat of the first deficient generation is placed back on an optimum raw diet after giving birth to a deficient litter, her next kittens, benefiting from her improved diet, are called Regenerating Kittens of the First Order.

Regenerating Kittens of the Second Order: These kittens are born to a cat of the second deficient generation and are placed on an optimum diet.

There are never more than three generations of deficient cats because of the third generation's inability to produce healthy, viable offspring. Consequently, there are no third or fourth orders of regenerating cats.

Chapter Two

THE RAW MEAT VERSUS COOKED MEAT
FEEDING EXPERIMENT

"The Effect of Heat-Processed Foods and Vitamin D Metabolized Milk on the Dentofacial Structures of Experimental Animals," "Heat Labile Factors Necessary for the Proper Growth and Development of Cats," "Clinical and Experimental Evidence of Growth Factors in Raw Milk," "The Influence of Heat Labile Factors on Nutrition in Oral Development and Health"

In this feeding experiment, one group of cats receives a diet of $^2/_3$ raw meat, $^1/_3$ raw milk, and cod liver oil. The second group receives $^2/_3$ cooked meat, $^1/_3$ raw milk, and cod liver oil. Comparisons are made between the two groups on the basis of their growth, skeletal development, dentofacial structures, and dental health, the calcium and phosphorus content of their femurs at death, their resistance to infections, their allergic sensitivity, and their reproductive efficiency (reproductive efficiency as used by Dr. Pottenger means the ability of the female cat to become pregnant, deliver, and nurse viable offspring).

GENERAL OBSERVATIONS

Raw Meat Group

The cats fed a diet of $^2/_3$ raw meat, $^1/_3$ raw milk, and cod liver oil show striking uniformity in their sizes and their skeletal developments. From generation to generation they maintain a regular, broad face with prominent malar and orbital arches, adequate nasal cavities, broad dental arches, and regular dentition. The configuration of the female skull is different from the male skull, and each sex maintains its distinct anatomical features. The membranes are firm and of good pink color with no evidence of infection or degenerative change. Tissue tone is excellent, and the fur of good quality with very little shedding noted. In the older cats, particularly the males engaging in fighting, the incisors are often missing, but inflammation and disease of the gums is seldom seen.

9

The calcium and phosphorus content of their femurs remains consistent, and their internal organs show full development and normal function. Over their life spans, they prove resistant to infections, to fleas, and to various other parasites, and show no signs of allergies. In general, they are gregarious, friendly, and predictable in their behavior patterns, and when thrown or dropped as much as 6 feet to test their coordination, they always land on their feet and come back for more "play." These cats reproduce one homogeneous generation after another, with the average weight of the kittens at birth being 119 grams. Miscarriages are rare, and litters average five kittens with the mother cat nursing her young without difficulty.

Cooked Meat Group

The cats fed a diet of $^2/_3$ raw meat, $^1/_3$ raw milk, and cod liver oil reproduce a heterogeneous strain of kittens, each kitten in a litter being different in size and skeletal pattern. When comparing the changes in configuration found in their X-rays, there are almost as many variations in the facial and dental structures of the second- and third-generation cats fed cooked meat as there are animals. Evidence of deficiencies is written so plainly on their faces that, with a little training, any observer can be almost certain that a given cat has been subjected to a deficient diet or that it comes from a line of cats that has suffered from deficient nutrition.

The long bones of cats fed cooked meat tend to increase in length and decrease in diameter, with the hind legs commonly increasing in length over the forelegs. The trabeculation (the internal structural mesh of the bones) becomes coarser and shows evidence of less calcium. In the third generation, some of the bones become as soft as rubber and a true condition of osteogenesis imperfecta is present.

Heart problems; nearsightedness and farsightedness; underactivity of the thyroid or inflammation of the thyroid gland; infections of the kidney, of the liver, of the testes, of the ovaries, and of the bladder; arthritis and inflammation of the joints; inflammation of the nervous system with paralysis and meningitis—all occur commonly in these cats fed cooked meat. A decrease in visceral volume is evidenced by the diminishing size of their thoracic and abdominal cavities. Frank infections of the bone appear regularly and often appear to be the cause of death. By the time the third deficient generation is born, the cats are so physiologically bankrupt that none survive beyond the sixth month of life, thereby terminating the strain.

A study of the microscopic sections of the lungs of second- and third-generation deficient cats show abnormal respiratory tissues. The lungs show hyperemia, some edema, and partial atelectasis, and the most deficient show bronchitis and pneumonitis. In several cases, a hypothyroid condition exists, with the thyroid gland showing scanty colloid and small acini, again not observable in cats fed raw meat.

Cats fed cooked meat show much more irritability. Some females are even dangerous to handle, and three are named Tiger, Cobra, and Rattlesnake because of their proclivity for biting and scratching. The males, on the other hand, are more docile, often to the point of being unaggressive, and their sex interest is slack or perverted. In essence, there is evidence of a role reversal with the female cats becoming the aggressors and the male cats becoming passive, as well as evidence of increasing abnormal activities between the same sexes. Such sexual deviations are not observed among the cats fed raw food.

Vermin and intestinal parasites abound. Skin lesions and allergies appear frequently and are progressively worse from one generation to the next. Pneumonia and empyema are among the principal causes of death in adult cats, and diarrhea followed by pneumonia takes a heavy toll on the kittens.

At autopsy, females fed cooked meat frequently present ovarian atrophy and uterine congestion, and the males often show failure in the development of active spermatogenesis. Abortion in pregnant females is common, running about 25 percent in the first deficient generation to about 70 percent in the second generation. Deliveries are generally difficult with many females dying in labor. The mortality rate of the kittens also is high, as the kittens are either born dead or are born too frail to nurse. Following delivery, a few mother cats steadily decline in health only to die from some obscure physiological exhaustion in about three months. Other cats show increasing difficulty with their pregnancies, and in many instances, fail to become pregnant. The average weight of the kittens born of mothers fed cooked meat is 100 grams, 19 grams less than the kittens nurtured on raw meat.

Figure 2.1 shows a cat that has been on a diet of cooked meat for over a year. She delivers six kittens, two of which she eats on the first day. She shows no inclination to care for the remaining. Upon examination, it is found that she is unable to nurse her kittens because her mammary glands present no evidence of preparation for lactation. The four kittens are placed on dropper feedings of cow's milk on the second day. Three die of diarrhea

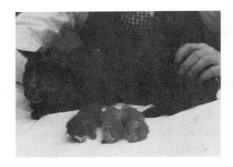 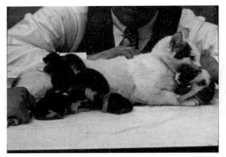

Fig. 2.1—Adult female cat 524. On cooked meat and raw milk for six months and during pregnancy. 1936 litter. Note dull eyes, poor fur. Three kittens, 4 days old, dead.

Fig 2.2—Adult female cat, one year old, on raw meat and milk. First litter in pens, 1936. Four kittens, 4 days old. Note full development and activity of kittens. Note smoothness and luster of fur. Inactive kitten, second from left, is kitten of cat 524.

on the third day. The fourth is placed with the lactating cat shown in Figure 2.2, but it dies on the fourth day in spite of every attempt on the part of the foster mother to care for it.

Figure 2.2 shows a mother fed raw food and her four kittens born the day before the ill-fated kittens above. The mother cat is 11 months old and has been fed raw meat, raw milk, and cod liver oil since the age of two months. She delivers six kittens, losing two on account of her failure to rupture the amniotic sac in time. She has large mammae and has no difficulties in nursing her young. Her kittens have broad faces and show excellent skeletal development.

Regenerating Cats

When cats of the first- and second-generation groups fed cooked meat are returned to a diet of raw meat, they are classified as regenerating animals of the first and second orders. Their progeny are then maintained on an optimum diet to measure the time needed to rebuild their health to that of the normal cats. It requires approximately four generations for either order to regenerate to a state of normal health. However, because of the lack of reproductive efficiency, very few deficient animals regain the normal health noted before deficiency was imposed on their line of cats.

Improvement in resistance to disease is noted in the second-generation regenerating cat, but allergic manifestations persist into the third generation. In the third generation, skeletal and soft tissue changes are still noticeable, but to a lesser degree; and by the fourth generation, most of the severe deficiency signs and symptoms disappear—but seldom completely.

One of the experiment's more startling discoveries is that, once a female cat is subjected to a deficient diet for a period of 12 to 18 months, her reproductive efficiency is so reduced that she is never again able to give birth to normal kittens. Even after three or four years of eating an optimum diet, her kittens still show signs of deficiency in skeletal and dental development. When her kittens are maintained on an optimum diet, a gradual reversal and regeneration takes place.

VARIATION—RAW MEAT AND COOKED MEAT ALTERNATED

In this experiment, one group of cats is fed raw meat, placed on a diet of cooked meat for six months, and then returned to a diet of raw meat. (The six-month exposure to cooked food is timed to correspond to the human teenage years.) When a female cat on this alternated diet becomes pregnant, her kittens exhibit some deficiency symptoms, although she may appear in good health. Her succeeding litters show irregularities that tend to lessen in intensity for the first two or three years of her reproductive life and then increase again. As long as her kittens receive the optimum raw diet, their health improves; however, when they are given cooked meat for a period of time, their resistance to disease greatly diminishes, only to improve when they are returned to the diet of raw meat. These cats fed a diet alternating between raw meat and cooked meat partially maintain their skeletal structures from generation to generation, but their calcification continues to diminish, and their reproductive efficiency is injured from the standpoints of the size and the vitality of their kittens and of the failure of their litters to conform to a homogeneous pattern.

Chapter Three

THE RAW MILK VERSUS COOKED MILK
FEEDING EXPERIMENT

"The Effect of Heat-Processed Foods and Metabolized Vitamin D Milk on the Dentofacial Structures of Experimental Animals," "Clinical and Experimental Evidence of Growth Factors in Raw Milk," "The Reciprocal Relationship of Soil, Plant and Animal," "Clinical Evidences of the Value of Raw Milk"

This feeding experiment involves four groups of cats. One group receives a diet of $2/3$ raw milk, $1/3$ raw meat, and cod liver oil. The other groups receive a diet of either $2/3$ pasteurized milk, $2/3$ evaporated milk or $2/3$ sweetened condensed milk, plus $1/3$ raw meat, and cod liver oil.

GENERAL OBSERVATIONS

The results of this experiment correspond to those of the raw meat versus cooked meat experiment. Animals on raw milk and raw meat reproduce homogeneous litters, and the usual causes of death are old age and injuries suffered in fighting. They are generally healthy animals with normal anatomic measurements and good resistance to disease. Their fur is of good quality with a notable sheen, and they show no signs of allergy.

The cats fed pasteurized milk as the principal item of their diet show skeletal changes and lessened reproductive efficiency, and their kittens present progressive constitutional and respiratory problems as is evident in the first-, second- and third-generation cats eating cooked meat.

Cats fed evaporated milk show even more damage than their pasteurized milk counterparts, but the most marked deficiencies occur among those fed sweetened condensed milk. The cats on sweetened condensed milk develop much heavier fat deposits and exhibit severe skeletal deformities. They show extreme irritability and nervously pace back and forth in their pens.

Table I reveals the effects of condensed milk, evaporated milk, pasteurized milk, and metabolized vitamin D milk on the life span of specific experimental animals.

TABLE I. MILK EXPERIMENT NUMBER IV

(Experiment to study effect of heat-processed milk in the development and longevity of cats fed one-third enough raw meat to maintain them and two-thirds the amount of food from milk. Note that the animals on the diet of metabolized vitamin D milk died within two months, but most litter mates survived the entire experiment. Start of experiment, Dec. 12, 1940; close of experiment, Aug. 13, 1941 [8 months].)

NUMBER AND ORDER	AGE AT BEGINNING OF EXPERIMENT	LENGTH OF LIFE AFTER EXPERIMENT BEGAN
Male	*Condensed Milk*	
*788 1 Re L1	$9^{1/2}$ months	8 months
749 1 Re L3	$7^{1/2}$ months	3 months
757 1 Re L3	$7^{1/2}$ months	8 months
Female		
644 Re	Adult	$4^{1/2}$ months
646 1 Re L1	1 year 7 months	$4^{1/2}$ months
506 Re	2 years 6 months	8 months
Male	*Evaporated Milk*	
789 1 Re L1	$9^{1/2}$ months	8 months
750 1 Re L3	$7^{1/2}$ months	$4^{1/2}$ months
760 1 Re L3	$7^{1/2}$ months	8 months
Female		
794 Re	Adult	$4^{1/2}$ months
693 1 Re L1	2 years	8 months
678 1 Re L2	1 year 4 months	$5^{3/4}$ months
Male	*Pasteurized Milk*	
790 1 Re L1	$9^{1/2}$ months	8 months
752 1 Re L3	$7^{1/2}$ months	2 months
761 1 Re L3	$7^{1/2}$ months	8 months
Female		
691 Re	2 years	8 months
569 1 Re L1	1 year 8 months	$2^{1/2}$ months
532 Re	3 years	8 months
Male	*Metabolized Vitamin D Milk*	
792 1 Re L1	$9^{1/2}$ months	1 month 22 days
753 1 Re L3	$7^{1/2}$ months	1 month 16 days
763 1 Re L3	$7^{1/2}$ months	1 month 11 days
Female		
533 Re	4 years	8 months
697 1 Re L1	$1^{1/2}$ years	8 months
694 Re	$5^{1/2}$ years	8 months

Males 788, 789, 790, 792—litter mates
Males 749, 750, 752, 753—litter mates
Males 757, 760, 761, 763—litter mates

*Explanation: 1 = First generation; Re = regenerating; L1 = first litter. Example: 1 Re L1 = First generation, regenerating, first litter. It is the first-generation, raw-meat animal born to a cat after it had been on a cooked-meat diet.

VARIATION—METABOLIZED VITAMIN D MILK

In this experiment, cats receive vitamin D milk (from cattle fed irradiated yeast) and raw meat. The male cats show osseous disturbances very like those on pasteurized milk, but the females appear unaffected. An interesting circumstance occurred in the males fed this milk. Young males did not live beyond the second month, and adult males died within ten months. There is a notable tendency for the calcium/phosphorus ratio to become unbalanced, approaching 2.5 to 1 as compared to a normal of 2 to 1. This tendency is accompanied by bone changes, including the development of rickets in some of the young animals. See Table II.

It is worth noting that natural cod liver oil, which is rich in vitamin D, does not appear to adversely affect the development of either the male or the female cats, but the metabolized vitamin D milk from cattle fed irradiated yeast is damaging to the males.

TABLE II. LONGEVITY OF CATS FED IRRADIATED VITAMIN D MILK

(Four litter-mate, well-developed male kittens fed raw meat, age 1½ months, were placed on two metabolized vitamin D milks—one from a certified farm where the cattle received green feed, and the other where cattle received dry feed. Note that the cattle fed the dry feed gave milk that produced rickets when fed to cats, in spite of the high amount of vitamin D present. The vitamin D irradiated milk was the sole source of food.)

	DIET	RICKETS	FIRST AND LAST WEIGHT	WEIGHT CHANGE	CALCIUM PHOSPHORUS RATIO	DATE AND CAUSE OF DEATH
Female 359	Raw meat control	0	605 1,145	+840	(2) Ca 13.27 P 6.72	Chloroformed 6/24/36
Male 360	Green feed, vitamin D milk	0	620 540	−80	(191) Ca 15.52 P 8.12	Pneumonia 6/16/36
Male 361	Green feed, vitamin D milk	0	580 501	−79	(202) Ca 15.86 P 7.85	Pneumonia 6/16/36
Male 362	Dry feed, vitamin D milk	Present	640 506	−134	(205) Ca 15.60 P 7.61	Pneumonia 6/15/36
Male 263	Dry feed, vitamin D milk	Present	700 537	−163	(216) Ca 17.71 P 7.27	Severe Rickets 6/15/36

Litter mates born March 1, 1936.
Experiment started April 15, 1936.
Milk was sole diet.

VARIATION—RAW MILK FROM COWS FED DRY FEED AND FROM COWS FED FRESH FEED

In the course of producing and marketing adrenal cortical extracts, we began noting that the adrenal glands being used differed greatly in their potency.* Seeking an explanation for this, we discovered that the glands of the highest potency came from cows and steers killed in Denver and those of the lowest potency came from cows and steers slaughtered in the Los Angeles area. Tracing this back, we learned that Denver animals were pastured on young, rapid-growing range grasses, but the Los Angeles animals were fed mostly dry feed consisting of molasses, cotton seed meal, beet pulp, orange pulp, grape pulp and other industrial by-products, field-dried alfalfa, and grain. We further learned that the reproductive efficiency of range cows is greater than dry feed lot cows and that a high rate of mortality exists among dry feed lot calves.

From this information, it appears logical to assume that dietary factors not only influence the potency of adrenal glands, but also influence the nutritive quality of cow's milk. Just as the adrenal hormones of cows fed on green pasture continually show a high concentration and potency, so their milk appears to have a high concentration of the growth activators necessary for their calves' healthy development; and just as the hormones of dry feed lot cows are of low concentration, so their milk appears deficient in the growth activators necessary for nurturing and supporting their young.

In comparing the experimental effects on cats of a diet including raw milk from cows fed fresh feed and those of a diet including raw milk from cows fed dry feed, we find that the cats fed raw milk from dry-feed cows show similar deficiencies as those fed pasteurized milk. Moreover, cats fed cooked meat, milk produced from dry-feed cattle, and cod liver oil always deliver deficient kittens and have trouble nursing, but cats fed a high-grade raw milk from cows grazing on green pasture or from cows fed freshly cut greens, cooked meat, and cod liver oil do better. The high-grade raw milk appears to lessen the deficiencies produced by the cooked meat. Conversely, cats fed dry-feed raw milk, raw meat, and cod liver oil deliver normal kittens and have adequate milk supplies. Here, the raw meat counters the deficiency in the dry-feed raw milk.

---

*As the text reflects Francis M. Pottenger's original writing, the "we" refers to him and his staff.

Chicken Industry

The same dry-feed versus fresh-feed findings hold true of the chicken industry.

Farm chickens get out and scratch for worms and eat green grasses and weeds. They lay eggs with hard shells and deep yellow yokes; and when these eggs are fertilized, they hatch husky, healthy chicks. In addition, farm chickens have supple skin, firm musculature, and almost twice as much calcium for a given weight of bone as mass-produced, hatchery chickens.

In contrast, hatchery chickens are housed in wire pens and fed various grains and other dry feeds. They lay eggs with thin shells and pale yokes; and when their eggs are fertilized, a large percentage fail to germinate. The hatchery chicken has thick skin, lax musculature, pale fat, soft flesh, and much smaller bones than the farm chicken.

In comparing the diets of farm and hatchery chickens and of range and dry feed lot cattle, we find that they all contain adequate amounts of fat, protein, carbohydrate, and minerals. *The difference lies in the presence or absence of fresh factors.* It is the fresh, raw factors in feed that appear to hold the balance between a healthy animal capable of reproducing healthy offspring and one that is unhealthy and has poor reproductive efficiency. Logically, the nutritional value of animal products such as milk and eggs depends on the nutritional value of the producing animal's diet. (See work of Oscar Erf, Chap. 10.)

VARIATION—GUINEA PIGS FED DRY FEED AND FRESH FEED

In this experiment, a group of guinea pigs is initially fed a diet of rolled and cracked grain with supplements of cod liver oil and field-dried alfalfa. Shortly, they show loss of hair, paralysis, and high litter mortality. Diarrhea, pneumonia, and other deficiency symptoms increase. When fresh-cut green feed (grass cut after sundown, sacked, and delivered before sunrise) is introduced into their diet, the guinea pigs show remarkable improvement. Infant mortality decreases, and the animals become huskier. No new cases of paralysis develop, and the alopecia lessens, though it does not disappear entirely. A few guinea pigs with severe diarrhea and loss of hair are allowed to run outside the pens to feed on growing grass and weeds. In less than 30 days, these foraging animals show even greater improvement than those receiving cut greens inside the pens. Their diarrhea stops; their hair returns with a soft, shiny, velvety texture; they heal and become well. When they are placed back inside the pens, they show no further signs of gastrointestinal upset or other ailments.

Looking for an explanation of this more dramatic improvement in the guinea pigs feeding on the fresh-growing grasses and weeds, we noticed that, when we put our arms inside the sacks of cut grass, the temperature inside was warmer than the temperature outside. It proved to range between 5 degrees and 30 degrees warmer. This suggests that the sacked, cut grass becomes semicooked by the time it reaches the guinea pigs and that important thermolabile substances are at least partly destroyed.

Chapter Four

THE EFFECT OF RAW AND COOKED FOOD ON THE DENTOFACIAL DEVELOPMENT OF CATS

"The Effect of Heat-Processed Foods and Metabolized Vitamin D Milk on the Dentofacial Structures of Experimental Animals," "The Influence of Heat Labile Factors on Nutrition in Oral Development and Health," "Nutritional Aspects of the Orthodontic Problem"

Normal Cats

The cats receiving a raw meat, raw milk diet maintain a regular broad face with prominent malar and orbital arches, adequate nasal cavities, broad dental arches, and regular dentition from generation to generation. The configuration of the female skull remains distinct from that of the male, and each maintains its normal facial outlines. The mucous membranes are firm and of good pink color, showing no evidence of infection or degenerative change. The teeth erupt without difficulty and remain basically free of decay. See Figures 4.1 and 4.2.

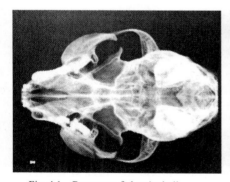 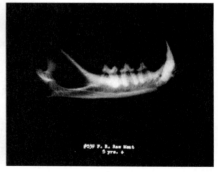

Fig. 4.1—Raw-meat-fed cat's skull.

Fig. 4.2—Lateral X-ray of half jaw of cat 539, showing a normal jaw structure, good distribution of trabeculae, well-developed condyle, and well-developed pterygoid process of the mandible. Alveolar crest of normal height; even distribution of teeth.

Deficient Cats

First Generation: Adult cats placed on a diet of cooked meat or pasteurized milk begin to show unhealthy conditions in their mouths within three to six months. A pregnant cat shows the changes more rapidly. These cats first present gingivitis followed by incrustation of salivary calculi, which continues to increase whether the cat is maintained on a deficient diet or returned to an optimum diet. As salivary deposits increase, their gums become spongy. This leads to infections and abscesses, which sometimes break through the lining of the cheek and drain outside. In three to five years, all the incisors and most of the molars are missing. The "fangs" or canine teeth prove the most resistant to abscesses and loss. Interestingly, no caries are noted in this first deficient generation of cats. See Figure 4.3.

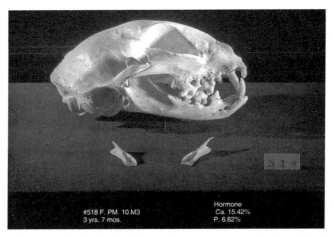

#518 F. PM. 10.M3
3 yrs. 7 mos.

Hormone
Ca. 15.42%
P. 6.62%

Fig. 4.3—First-generation female cat 518, nursed one month, on a cooked-meat diet for three years, three months. She was then placed on the pasteurized milk experiment and died three months later. Note flattening of the entire skull with poor development of the condylar fossae. Distance from the zygomatic arch to the lower border of the mandible is lesser in the posterior jaw than the anterior in the region of the premolar teeth. There is well-developed paradentosis with vertical atrophy, poor distribution of trabeculae, and erosion of the condyle. Root resorption present in both upper and lower teeth.

Second Generation: In the second generation of cats fed cooked food, the newborn deficient kittens show irregular development of the contours of the skull cap and a narrowing of the malar and orbital arches. The latter become incomplete as deficiency progresses. Most of the cats show longer and narrower faces with a retraction in the middle third due to diminished development of the zygomatic arch and diminished closure of the frontal sinuses. Failure in the lateral movement of the face causes material narrowing of the mandible and maxillary portions so that there is insufficient room for a complete set of teeth to descend into place; and recessive or protruding mandibles are common, causing underbites and overbites. See Figures 4.6, 4.7, and 4.8.

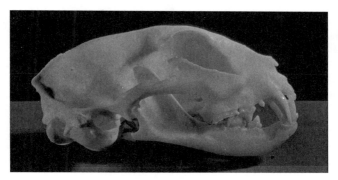

Fig 4.6—Second-generation male cat 513, second litter, fed cooked meat. Note apparently good skull except for incomplete orbital arch, resorption of the condyle, and the pulling up of the posterior portion of the mandible in comparison with the anterior portion.

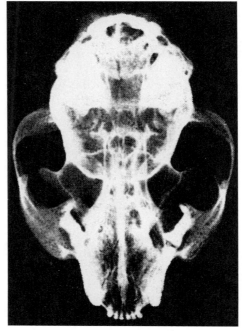

Fig. 4.7—X-ray of basal view of skull of second-generation male cat 513, as in Fig. 4.6. Note lack of development of orbital arch and osteoporosis.

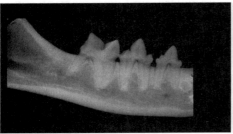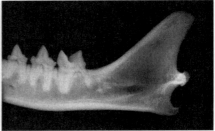

Fig. 4.8—X-rays of mandible of male cat 513, as in Fig. 4.6. Note extreme osteoporosis, with almost complete loss of trabeculae and failure in development of the heads of the condyles.

There is frequent delay in the loss of the deciduous teeth, and therefore, permanent teeth do not erupt at a regular time as they do in the cats fed raw food. Their eruption is often accompanied by bleeding gums, runny noses, fevers, and prostration, as opposed to normal cats that have teeth without problems. The primary teeth are usually smaller and more irregular in size and in shape than those of normal kittens. This is particularly true of the central incisors, but also is true of the canines, premolars, and molars.

Where the canine teeth are quite resistant to deficiency in the first generation, active root absorption occurs in the second generation with softening of the base of the apices and loosening of the teeth. Frequently, the canines fall out before the molars. Absence of teeth, especially the incisors, is quite common. As the jaw does not expand or widen to make room for the permanent teeth, these teeth show considerable crowding, twisting, and impaction. See Figure 4.9.

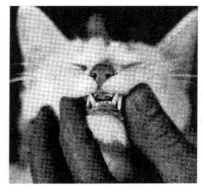

Fig 4.9—Female kitten, age 12 months, litter mate of kitten in Fig. 4.10, fed table scraps until 10 months of age. Note imperfect alignment of teeth.

The permanent teeth show greater irregularity in their size and alignment than the deciduous teeth. Marked retraction of the mandible with failure in calcification causes poor bony support for the teeth. As in the first generation of deficiency, gums are spongy and abscesses develop. An interesting finding is that root resorption occurs more commonly among cats fed a diet of heat-processed milk than among those fed cooked meat.

Third Generation: The degenerative changes in the skull and mouth grow more pronounced in the third generation of cats fed cooked food. The frontal sinuses and zygomatic arch show little development, which allows for further retraction of the middle third of the face. The skull of the second-generation deficient adult is smaller than that of the first deficient generation of the same age. The skull of the third generation is materially smaller than that of the second generation. However, there are some variations. Some kittens have larger than normal brain cases with smaller than normal faces, and these animals have a relatively poor forward projection of the face as a whole. At times there is a marked tendency for the configuration of the skull in both males and females to approach the shape of the normal animal of the opposite sex.

In these third-generation deficient cats, the bones are very fine with scarcely enough structure to hold the skull together. The teeth are smaller and much more irregular in size, shape, and alignment, and when the permanent teeth erupt, the cats are frequently prostrate. In some of these deficient kittens, the failure of the anterior movement of the jaw is so great that the posterior molars, instead of being embedded in the corpus of the mandible, remain in the ramus; and the crown of the teeth, instead of being parallel to the floor of the mouth, is perpendicular to it—a description of impacted wisdom teeth.

Kittens in which deficiency is established by an inadequate diet show stigmata throughout their lives. If deficient kittens are allowed to live in the open and to feed upon rats, mice, birds, gophers, and other food natural to the cat, they will show a certain degree of correction in their deficiencies.

Two litter mates offer a good comparative example of the improvement possible by a natural diet. The mother of these two kittens is a deficient animal eating cooked food. One of the litter mates is kept in a pen on a similar deficient diet until approximately ten months of age; the other, at five weeks of age, is forced to forage in the wilds. The penned kitten shows marked dental deformity; the foraging kitten shows the effects of

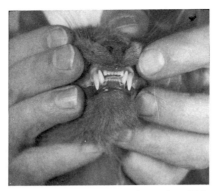

Fig. 4.10—Female kitten, age 12 months, forced to forage for self from the age of 4 to 6 weeks. Note regular alignment of teeth.

its deficient history, but reveals major correction in the alignment of its teeth and in its general physiological stability. See Figure 4.10.

The improvement in the foraging kitten is probably caused by its better diet, but also by the exercise it received eating its hunted prey with all the ripping, tearing, and chewing involved to work its jaw and facial muscles. Even though the occlusion of its teeth is good, the teeth are not of normal size.

If proper nutrition and exercise are absent when facial structures are developing, dentition always suffers. The kitten kept on a deficient diet for 10 months has an inadequate jaw with crowded, irregular, and poorly aligned teeth.

The deficient stigmata persist in the two litter mates, and both die at 14 months as a result of pregnancy.

Regenerating Cats

In the regenerating cats, skull development is still deficient in the second generation with a universal malalignment of teeth. The third generation shows marked improvement, and in the fourth generation, an occasional cat shows normal skull and dental development.

Chapter Five

THE EFFECT OF RAW AND COOKED FOOD ON THE CALCIUM AND PHOSPHORUS CONTENT OF BONES

"Deficient Calcification Produced by Diet: Experimental and Clinical Consideration," "Reciprocal Relationship of Soil, Plant and Animal," "The Influence of Heat Labile Factors on Nutrition in Oral Development and Health"

The calcium and phosphorus content as well as the weight and size of the femurs of normal and deficient cats are determined at death. The kittens of mother cats on raw food and on cooked food all prove to have approximately the same amount of calcium and phosphorus at birth. Quite often, this is within two to three percent of that found in the mothers. See Table III.

After the first two weeks, a marked depletion of the calcium and phosphorus content of the femurs occurs in the kittens. This corresponds to the period of the greatest growth. However, within two months, the bones of the kittens nurtured on raw food are approaching normal in respect to these salts, but those of the kittens on cooked food lag behind. This effect is still more pronounced in the second and third deficient generations; that is, the bones of the second- and third-generation deficient kittens on cooked food are markedly deficient in calcium and phosphorus. Kittens on raw food have from two to three times as much calcium and phosphorus in their bones. See Tables IV and V.

TABLE III. CALCIUM AND PHOSPHORUS CONTENT OF FEMURS OF NEWBORN KITTENS AND THEIR MOTHERS

	CAT NUMBER	TYPE OF CAT DIET	SEX	AGE	WEIGHT OF CAT (GRAMS)	WEIGHT OF FEMUR (GRAMS)	CALCIUM IN FEMUR (%)	PHOSPHORUS IN FEMUR (%)
A. Kittens:	a	Raw	—	1 day	—	0.1091	10.06	6.02
	b	Raw	—	5 days	129	0.1305	12.23	5.78
	c	Raw	F	5 days	115	0.1451	14.25	7.15
	d	Cooked	—	1 day	—	0.1330	11.92	6.15
	e	Cooked	F	1 day	112	0.0829	10.79	5.49
B. Mother Cats:	a1	Raw	F	13 mos.	3200	7.74	10.04	4.83
	c1	Raw	F	14 mos.	1957	8.09	12.43	5.60
	d1	Cooked	F	6 yrs.	4600	10.78	14.00	6.35

Mother of corresponding kitten indicated by subletter.

TABLE IV. CALCIUM AND PHOSPHORUS CONTENT OF FEMURS OF KITTENS FED RAW FOOD

CAT NUMBER	SEX	AGE	WEIGHT OF CAT (GRAMS)	WEIGHT OF FEMUR (GRAMS)	Weight of Femur BODY WEIGHT (%)	CALCIUM (%)	PHOSPHORUS (%)
1	—	1 day	—	0.1091	—	10.06	6.02
2	—	5 days	129	0.1305	0.10	12.23	5.78
3	F	5 days	115	0.1451	0.12	14.25	7.15
4	—	3 weeks	—	0.75	—	5.31	2.26
5	M	5 weeks	335	0.98	0.28	7.04	3.89
6	F	5 weeks	393	1.06	0.27	7.50	3.74
7	M	5 weeks	377	0.79	0.21	10.59	5.28
8	F	8 weeks	965	4.77	0.49	4.73	2.25
9	M	8 weeks	977	5.21	0.53	5.97	2.85
10	F	8 weeks	715	4.25	0.59	6.48	3.10
11	F	12 weeks	1085	5.63	0.52	7.64	3.66
12	F	12 weeks	800	5.67	0.71	8.55	4.21
13	F	12 weeks	1062	5.87	0.55	8.61	4.09
14	M	12 weeks	1277	6.95	0.54	8.69	3.95
15	F	12 weeks	900	4.89	0.54	8.83	4.08
16	F	12 weeks	1300	6.17	0.62	9.45	4.31
17	M	12 weeks	1275	5.01	0.39	11.59	4.93
18	M	14 weeks	1117	4.53	0.41	15.03	7.35
19	F	10 mos.	1503	9.37	0.62	11.60	5.17
20	M	13.5 mos.	2732	8.48	0.31	12.40	6.02
Averages			1008	4.23		9.48	4.55
	C/P 2.08						

TABLE V. CALCIUM AND PHOSPHORUS CONTENT OF FEMURS OF DEFICIENT KITTENS

CAT NUMBER	SEX	AGE	WEIGHT OF CAT (GRAMS)	WEIGHT OF FEMUR (GRAMS)	Weight of Femur BODY WEIGHT (%)	CALCIUM (%)	PHOSPHORUS (%)
1	F	1 day	112	0.0829	0.074	10.79	5.49
2	—	1 day	—	0.1330	—	11.92	6.15
3	—	3 weeks	261	0.75	0.28	5.32	2.53
4	F	7 weeks	310	1.84	0.59	5.14	2.41
5	M	7 weeks	261	0.97	0.26	6.76	3.24
6	F	8 weeks	400	1.93	0.48	4.49	2.42
7	M	9 weeks	565	2.91	0.51	3.19	1.61
8	M	9 weeks	514	2.83	0.55	3.37	1.73
9	F	9 weeks	434	1.94	0.45	6.27	2.29
10	M	12 weeks	335	2.15	0.64	4.32	2.20
11	F	12 weeks	523	3.28	0.62	3.51	1.79
12	M	14 weeks	1120	5.25	0.46	2.88	1.53
13	M	14 weeks	610	4.39	0.72	4.12	1.84
14	M	15 weeks	890	6.31	0.71	3.95	1.73
15	M	16 weeks	730	5.29	0.72	2.44	1.24
16	F	16 weeks	885	2.65	0.29	7.45	3.64
17	F	16 weeks	915	4.94	0.54	6.74	3.22
18	M	18 weeks	915	4.24	0.49	4.80	2.03
19	F	8.5 mos.	1009	2.85	0.28	4.77	2.42
20	F	14.5 mos.	1335	5.97	0.45	8.52	4.22
Averages			638	3.35		5.53	2.63
	C/P 2.63/1						

28

In Tables IV and V, the kittens are maintained on the respective diets of their mothers. The mothers on cooked meat are fed this diet at least six months before conception and throughout pregnancy. The ages of the 20 kittens nurtured on raw meat and 20 kittens nurtured on cooked meat range from 1 day to 14.5 months. The marked superiority of the kittens nurtured on raw meat as to weight of body and of femur is evident. The average body weight is 1008 grams for the kittens fed raw meat and 638 for the kittens fed cooked meat; the average weight of the femurs is 4.23 grams for the animals fed raw meat and 3.35 for those fed cooked meat. The average calcium content of the animals fed raw meat is 9.48 percent and 5.53 percent for those fed cooked meat. The average phosphorus content is 4.55 and 2.63, respectively. The average calcium/phosphorus ratio is 2.08/1 for the kittens fed raw meat and 2.63/1 for the kittens fed cooked meat. The higher calcium/phosphorus ratio in cats fed cooked meat is found in other studies.

When the experiment is repeated using milk as the test food, there is an equally profound change in the bones of the animals.

The percent of calcium in the bones of kittens fed raw and cooked food is plotted on the abscissa, with logarithm of age as the ordinate. See Figure 5.1. Kittens show a variability with age. It is to be noted that the peaks and dips are comparable in the two curves; each of the major dips corresponds to periods of eruption of teeth.

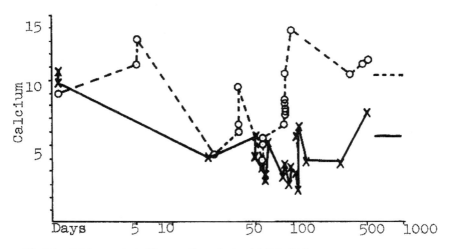

Fig. 5.1—Calcium content of femurs of raw-food and deficient kittens.

Analysis of the femurs of normal cats shows that the total amount of calcium in the fresh bone is approximately twice that of the phosphorus. The calcium in the femurs of normal adult cats with healthy parentage ranges between 12 and 17 percent, and the phosphorus ranges between 6 and 8.5 percent. The calcium content of the femur of the normal second-generation kitten, up to one year of age, falls between 8 and 12 percent. The deficient kitten of the second generation, up to one year of age, falls between 3.5 and 7 percent. The third-generation deficient cat may fall to the remarkable low of 1.5 to 3 percent of calcium. See Figure 5.2.

In Table VI, eighteen adult cats comparable in size, background, and general development are studied. Of the twelve fed raw meat and six fed cooked meat, the average weight of those fed raw meat is 2309 grams and 2253 for those fed cooked meat. The average weight of the femurs of the cats fed raw meat is 9.05 and 9.42 for those on cooked meat. The average calcium is 14.98 percent and 13.10 percent, respectively, and the average phosphorus content is 6.91 percent and 6.26 percent. The calcium/phosphorus ratio is constant at 2.1/1 and 2.09/1.

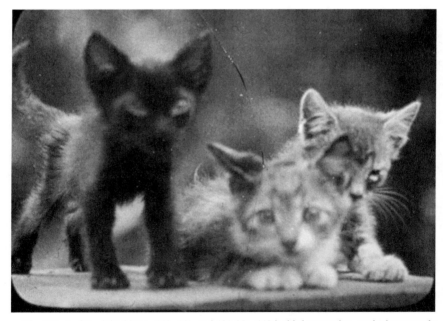

Fig. 5.2—Left to right, kittens 448, 461, and 481. No. 448 is third generation, cooked-meat male, first litter, age 2 months, 3 weeks. Ca 4.32; P 2.20. No. 461 is regenerating first order, second litter, female, age 2½ months. Ca 3.51; P 1.79. No. 481 is second-generation cooked-meat female, age 1¾ months. Ca 5.14; P 2.41.

TABLE VI. CALCIUM AND PHOSPHORUS CONTENT OF FEMURS OF ADULT CATS

CAT NUMBER	NORMAL OR DEFICIENT	SEX	WEIGHT OF CAT (GRAMS)	WEIGHT OF FEMUR (GRAMS)	*Weight of Femur* BODY WEIGHT (%)	CALCIUM IN FEMUR (%)	PHOSPHORUS IN FEMUR (%)
1	N	M	2947	11.44	0.39	11.22	5.26
2	N	F	1503	9.37	0.62	11.60	5.17
3	D	F	1531	5.14	0.33	11.74	5.86
4	D	F	2370	10.47	0.44	11.80	5.55
5	D	F	1490	6.51	0.43	12.99	6.38
6	N	M	2745	12.40	0.45	13.25	6.39
7	D	M	3120	15.40	0.49	13.36	6.73
8	N	M	1025	3.78	0.36	13.70	6.94
9	D	F	—	10.78	—	14.00	6.35
10	N	F	3300	12.29	0.37	14.30	6.66
11	D	F	2754	8.24	0.30	14.70	6.70
12	N	M	—	11.26	—	15.49	7.31
13	N	M	2390	7.80	0.26	15.67	8.15
14	N	F	1950	6.86	0.35	16.08	7.50
15	N	F	2295	9.58	0.42	16.40	7.92
16	N	F	1285	6.16	0.48	16.72	8.00
17	N	F	2650	8.39	0.31	17.02	8.14
18	N	F	3312	9.28	0.28	18.37	6.25
Averages	N		2309	9.05		14.98	6.91
	D		2253	9.42		13.10	6.26
	N	C/P 2.1					
	D	C/P 2.09					

Deficient cats on cooked meat and heat-processed milk reveal a decrease in the diameter of their bones, but their long bones tend to increase in length. By the third generation, these bones are soft like sponge rubber. They show spontaneous fractures on the slightest provocation; however, the fractures usually heal. Epiphyseal slips and injuries to the vertebrae are common. The bones of the mandible are just as soft as the other bones, and the teeth can be easily moved by the slightest touch of the finger.

Just as the calcium apparently diminishes progressively from the first through the second and the third generations of deficient cats, so there is a concomitant increase in the porosity of the bones. This is revealed through X-rays of the zygomatic arch. The trabecular structures become increasingly coarse. See Figures 5.3 and 5.4.

The first deficient generation shows trabeculation with the fineness of a silk scarf, that of the second generation is similar to a plain cotton handkerchief and that of the third generation is more like mosquito netting. Just as these three deficient structures vary in their mesh, so they vary in their ability to provide support.

When cats have excellent calcification through their growing years, up to the time of the closure of the epiphyses of the long bones, they have an excellent start in life. Those that show low calcification during their early years of life are less able to stand the usual stresses and strains ahead.

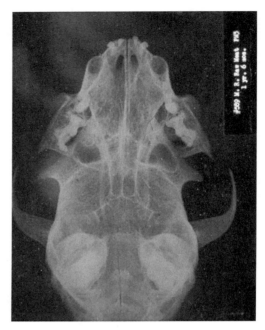

Fig. 5.3—X-ray of base of skull of regenerating male cat 589. Note lack of orbital and zygomatic arches and marked osteoporosis.

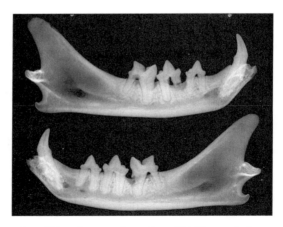

Fig. 5.4—X-ray of mandibles of regenerating male cat 589. Note marked osteoporosis and atrophy of the alveolar processes with small condyle head and poorly developed pterygoid process.

Chapter Six

ALLERGIES AND THYROID DEFICIENCY

"Nonspecific Methods for the Treatment of Allergic States," "The Influence of Heat Labile Factors on Nutrition in Oral Development and Health," "Effect of Heat-Processed Foods and Metabolized Vitamin D Milk on the Dentofacial Structures of Experimental Animals"

Normal cats on a diet of raw food and cod liver oil show no evidence of allergy or hypothyroidism; and their offspring, generation after generation, show no evidence of allergy or hypothyroidism. The incidence of these deficiency problems corresponds with the introduction of cooked foods.

Allergies

In giving cats cooked meat and milk, they develop all kinds of allergies. They sneeze, wheeze, and scratch. They are irritable, nervous, and do not purr. The first deficient generation of allergic cats produce second-generation kittens with greater incidence of allergies, and by the third generation, the incidence is almost 100 percent. When second-generation allergic animals are bred, after being returned to an optimum diet of raw food, their allergic symptoms begin to diminish, and by the fourth generation, some cats show no evidence of allergy. See Table VII.

One allergic cat reveals a condition analogous to the human disease pruritis ani, intense itching around the anus. In seeking relief, this animal rubs most of the fur off its buttocks, and its physical antics leave little doubt about its extreme discomfort. When milk is removed from the cat's diet, the allergic symptom immediately clears, revealing its specific allergen. Milk allergies prove common among second- and third-generation deficient cats and their regenerating counterparts.

One kitten develops asthma. Unfortunately, the animal dies before it is fully evaluated and before treatment is initiated. Apparently, this case of asthma is the first to be reported in the research literature.

33

TABLE VII. ALLERGIES IN KITTENS

	SECOND GEN. RAW				THIRD GEN. RAW				SECOND GEN. COOKED				THIRD GEN. COOKED				REGENERATING FIRST ORDER				REGENERATING SECOND ORDER			
	Litters	Total Number of Kittens	Allergic	Nonallergic	Litters	Total Number of Kittens	Allergic	Nonallergic	Litters	Total Number of Kittens	Allergic	Nonallergic	Litters	Total Number of Kittens	Allergic	Nonallergic	Litters	Total Number of Kittens	Allergic	Nonallergic	Litters	Total Number of Kittens	Allergic	Nonallergic
1936	2	7	0	7													2	8	6	2				
1937	3	11	0	11					3	14	5	9					4	17	13	4				
1938	7	24	0	24	1	3	0	3	4	13	4	9	1	3	2	1	3	13	3	10	2	6	0	6
1939	2	8	2	6	1	3	0	3	4	10	5	5	2	9	9	0	11	36	14	22	1	5	0	5
Total	14	50	2	48	1	3	0	3	11	37	14	23	3	12	11	1	20	74	36	38	3	11	0	11
Allergies (%)	4.0				0				37.8				91.6				48.6				0			

187 Kittens

All were 3 weeks of age or older.

Deficient cats were produced by feeding cooked-meat carcass as the major part of the diet. "Second generation raw" refers to kittens born to female cats in the pens that had been on raw meat all of their life in the pens. "Second generation raw" refers to kittens of the second generation maintained all their lives on raw meat. It is possible that two of the kittens in 1939 may have been born to mothers that had been deficient when brought into pens. "Third generation raw" refers to kittens of the second generation maintained all their lives on raw meat. "Second generation cooked" refers to kittens born to female cats maintained while in the pens on cooked meat and all during their pregnancy. "Third generation cooked" refers to the kitten of a second-generation cat fed cooked meat. Regeneration cats of "First Order" refers to kittens born to second-generation cats fed cooked meat after they had been returned to the raw-meat diet for at least one year and the pregnancy. Regenerating cats of the "Second Order" refers to kittens of the regenerating kittens of the First Order.

34

The intestinal tracts of the allergic cats prove particularly remarkable at autopsy. Measurements of the length of the gastrointestinal tracts of several hundred normal and deficient adult cats are compared. The measurement starts at the epiglottis and includes the esophagus, the stomach, duodenum, jejunum, and the colon to the rectum. In the average normal cat, the intestinal tract is approximately 48 inches long; in some of the allergic cats, the intestinal tracts measure as long as 72 to 80 inches. These elongated tracts lack tissue tone and elasticity.

Hypothyroidism

Thyroid deficiency produces marked disturbances in osseous development. An important physiologic factor in determining the bone development of infants, and later of adults, is the potency of the maternal thyroid. A disturbance in the thyroid function of the mother and/or of her ancestors shows in the anatomy of her young. Our diagnosis of thyroid deficiency in the female cat is based (1) on physical characteristics of her kittens, such as prominent frontal area of the skull, small teeth, retracted lower jaw, and failure of the anterior development of the face; and (2) on pathological examination of the thyroid tissue upon death.

Thyroid is a hormone known to pass from the mother into her milk and thus into her offspring. Use of supplementary thyroid in the diet of a nursing mother may produce symptoms of hyperthyroidism in her young. Among the nursing mother cats on a diet of raw meat and raw milk, there are no incidences of hypothyroidism among the kittens. Among the nursing mothers on cooked diets, there is a significant number of kittens with thyroid deficiency.

Figure 6.1 compares a kitten born of a thyroid-deficient mother with kittens born of mothers fed raw meat and cooked meat. Cat A (on the right) is a typically healthy male from healthy parents eating raw meat. He has a large skull, large bones, a large thorax, a large, long body, and relatively short legs. His dental arches are broad, and he has excellent teeth that are regular and well spaced.

Cat B (on the left) is born of a mother with a deficient thyroid. The mother has been on a raw-food diet for a year preceding his birth; however, during the time she was nursing her previous litter, she developed an abscess, which was diagnosed as a thyroid abscess by the character of some necrotic tissue obtained from the wound. This diagnosis was confirmed at autopsy. Though Cat B is approximately the same age as Cat A, he shows

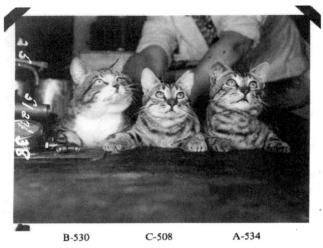

| B-530 | C-508 | A-534 |

Fig. 6.1—Left to right, male kittens 530, 508, and 534, all 18 months of age. No. 530, regenerating, first order, first litter, hypothyroid. Note failure in development of orbital and malar arches. No. 508, second-generation, first litter, kitten fed cooked meat. Note smallness of head, retraction of mandible, and failure in development of orbital and malar arches. No. 434, raw-meat cat.

markedly inferior development. There is a failure in the development of his face so that his teeth are crowded and narrow. His skull is smaller, his thorax smaller in diameter, his body shorter, and his legs longer than those of Cat A. All his soft tissues are inferior, meaning that their color is pale rather than red, that their elasticity is poor, that the muscle tone is poor, and that the fat is watery and white. As is typical of cats from hypothyroid mothers, he shows a much lower percentage of calcium and phosphorus in his femurs.

Cat C (middle) is an animal born of a mother fed cooked meat and kept on cooked meat all his life. He has a small skull, very narrow dental arch, irregular dentition, small body, and long legs. He is functionally sterile, and all his soft tissues are of very inferior quality.

A general finding in The Cat Study is that a correlation can be made between hypothyroidism in deficient cats and their lessened reproductive efficiency. Of the second-generation deficient male cats, 83 percent prove to be functionally sterile on pathological examination; that is, they exhibit no spermatozoa. Fifty-three percent of the females show underdeveloped and infantile ova.

As an example of the bizarre conditions that can be produced by long use of cooked food and by thyroid deficiency, the following kitten's history is interesting. The mother of this kitten is fed cooked meat for 18 months, placed on raw meat, and bred immediately. As soon as she delivers, she is put back on cooked food. During the nursing period, she develops a thyroid abscess, which is confirmed at autopsy. Of the four kittens born, two die within six weeks, one dies in three months, and the kitten in this example dies in eight months.

This kitten is named Streamlined because of her peculiar appearance. Her legs are bowed, her spine is distorted, and she develops a pot belly, which nearly reaches the ground. She has a wizened appearance, and when eight months old, she has the stature of a six-week-old kitten. About three months before death, Streamlined shows signs of paralysis in the left hind leg, which increases in severity until all legs become involved; one week before death, she has several convulsive seizures.

Her weight at death is 1009 grams. Postmortem examination reveals an underdeveloped animal with marked rickets, curvature of the spine, and a rachitic rosary of the ribs. The bladder is enormous, measuring 2.5 x 3.5 x 1 inch, and contains 110 cubic centimeters of urine. The urine accounts for more than 10 percent of the cat's weight. The bladder has pushed the intestines to the right side of the abdominal cavity to reveal a greatly enlarged colon. The femurs are soft and spongy and contain almost no cortex. Analysis of one of them shows that it contains 4.77 percent calcium and 2.42 percent phosphorus. This is 60 percent below normal for the age of the cat.

Chapter Seven

SUMMARY OF FINDINGS OF THE CAT STUDY

"Nutritional Aspects of the Orthodontic Problem," "Heat Labile Factors Necessary for the Proper Growth and Development of Cats," "Clinical Significance of the Osseous System," "Clinical Evidence of the Value of Raw Milk," "The Effect of Heat-Processed Foods and Metabolized Vitamin D Milk on the Dentofacial Structures of Experimental Animals"

On controlled experimental diets, we have been able to bring about developmental failure in cats. We have shown that allergic manifestations and dental disturbances comparable to those seen in human beings result from changes in food preparation.

The normal, wild cat subsists upon rodents, birds, reptiles, insects, fish, and a small amount of vegetation and maintains regular features and normal functions generation after generation. Ordinary house cats, living a semiwild life, also maintain regular features and functions generation after generation. In contrast, cats that are prevented from hunting, subjected to a life of ease, and fed prepared, cooked foods show tendencies toward maldevelopment.

In one experimental study, we compare two groups of cats on a base diet of raw milk and cod liver oil. The only difference in their food intake is that one group receives cooked meat and the other raw meat. The meat consists of viscera, muscle, and bone, and the cooked meat is prepared as if for human consumption. Comparisons of the two groups show many differences in development.

We find animals that receive raw meat show consistent facial development and normal dentition. Even so, these animals are not quite as perfect structurally as animals that forage and obtain their own natural foods. We also find the converse to be true. Those kittens that receive cooked meat instead of raw develop all types of malformations of the face, jaws, and teeth.

Adult cats that forage until they reach their maximum development and are then placed on a diet of cooked meat show little, if any, change in the contour of their skulls. An occasional animal might lose its teeth as a result of extensive decalcification and pyorrhea. When the well-developed cats are put on the cooked-meat diet and are allowed to become pregnant, their kittens' skulls show marked variations from the normal, no two have identical configuration. These changes occur in spite of ample food intake, and once such deficiencies are produced and maintained by a faulty diet, they become progressively worse through the second and third generations.

Differences in the effects of raw and cooked food appear in the weights of newborn kittens. During a three-year period, 63 living kittens born of parents fed raw food have an average weight of 119 grams at birth; and 47 kittens born of parents fed cooked food have an average weight of 100 grams. There are four dead kittens born in the group fed raw food and sixteen in the group fed cooked food.

The following offers a specific example of weight variations caused by changes in diet. One cat fed cooked food produces a litter of four kittens whose average weight is 77 grams. She is then placed on a raw-food diet, and her litter for the next year consists of five kittens with an average birth weight of 116 grams, and the following year (still on a diet of raw food), the litter consists of three kittens with an average weight of 137 grams.

The opposite result may be produced by taking a mother cat that has been on a diet of raw food and placing her on a diet of cooked food. In the case of one cat, her litter consists of five kittens with an average weight of 105 grams; the following year her litter consists of six kittens with an average weight of 91 grams.

The cats fed cooked food may produce a premature or full-term litter of stillborn kittens. One cat proves unable to deliver her kittens even after 72 hours of labor. If a mother cat is kept on cooked food for more than two years, she usually dies during delivery. Delivery complications such as these have not been found in cats placed on raw food.

When deficiency is produced in kittens, it cannot be reversed even under intense therapy. A well-developed cat can be maintained in a healthy state on deficient food if thyroid and adrenal hormones are added to her diet. A deficient kitten, even if given raw food, thyroid, and adrenal hormones, does not appear to become a normal cat.

One of the earliest defects noticed in the cats on cooked food is poor dentofacial development. Defects include: (1) a lessening of the anterior-posterior and transverse diameters of the dental arch; (2) an apparent alteration of the angle of the corpus of the mandible to the ramus; (3) an apparent failure in the anterior development of the forward movement of the face;

(4) a lessening in the development of the frontal sinuses; and (5) an increase in the angle formed by the roof of the mouth and the base of the brain.

The temporary teeth of both cats fed cooked foods and those fed raw foods seem well developed; however, when the permanent incisors displace the temporary ones, the cats on cooked food usually develop three or four irregularly spaced, uneven, crowded incisors instead of the usual six. This is true of both the upper and lower jaws. Decrease in the size and increase in irregularity of their teeth leads to malalignment and poor occlusion.

Diet definitely affects the mineralization of the bones. Analysis of the femurs at autopsy discloses that the calcium content of bones diminishes progressively from the first deficient generation to the third, ranging between 12 and 17 percent in the first generation to between 1.5 to 3 percent in the third. Phosphorus content of the bones also diminishes proportionately with deficiency. Deficient cats may have a longer shaft with a thinner than normal cortex. Their bones may be soft, spongy, and porous and show an apparent hyperplasia of the connective tissue cells in the bone marrow with lessening of the density of the bony trabeculae. These animals may show varying degrees of anemia. Disturbances of mineralization are transmitted from an afflicted mother cat to her offspring in an intensified form.

Deficient cats exhibit progressive allergic symptoms from generation to generation. They show most of the common respiratory, gastrointestinal and constitutional problems as well as various skin disorders. Their fur shows inferior quality, and their dispositions are much more nervous and irritable than those of normal cats. Hypothyroidism is prevalent and contributes to marked disturbances in the osseous development of some deficient cats and to apparent disturbances in their reproductive efficiency.

Cats can be so reduced in vitality by just one year of a diet considered adequate for human consumption that it may take them from two to three years to recover from the injury, if they can recover at all. If mother cats produce normal, healthy kittens, much can be done either to maintain their state of health or to reduce it to one of deficiency during the normal nursing period. The deficiency produced in a nursing kitten with healthy lineage cannot match the deficiency produced in a kitten born of a deficient mother during the nursing period. Milk produced by a deficient mother lacks the nutrients necessary for her kittens' normal growth and development, and its deficiency in these nutrients reinforces the deficiency already present in her kittens at birth. On the other hand, if such deficient kittens are given adequate feedings during the nursing period, much can be done to improve their general condition. It is our overall experience that any female cat that cannot nurse is deficient, just as any female cat that has too much milk is deficient.

The elements in raw food that activate and support growth and development in the young appear easily altered and destroyed by heat processing and oxidation. What are these vital elements? Their nature is not known at this time. We do know that ordinary cooking denatures proteins, rendering them less easily digested. Probably certain albuminoids and globulins are physiologically destroyed. All tissue enzymes are heat labile and so are destroyed. Vitamin C and some members of the B complex are injured by the process of cooking, and minerals are made less soluble by altering their physiochemical state. It is possible that the alteration of the physiochemical state of foods may be all that is necessary to make them deficient for the maintenance of healthy cats.

Now, how about humans?

Which Are Girls and Which Are Boys?

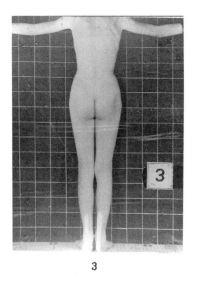

1

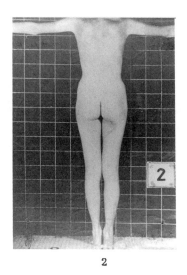

2

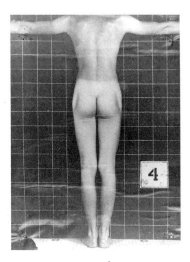

3

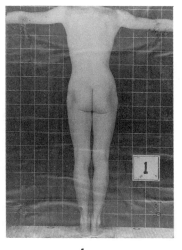

4

ANSWER: Numbers 1 and 4 are boys, numbers 2 and 3 are girls. Ages are between 15 and 17 years.

Part Two

Human Nutrition

Chapter Eight

HUMAN NUTRITION

"Which Are Girls and Which Are Boys?" "Does Social Practice Alter Man's Nutrition?" "Dietary Rehabilitation of the Malnourished," "Metabolic Factors of Development as Related to Physical Fitness"

The pictures on page 43 were shown at one of the American Medical Association Conventions. Physicians, nurses, and educators participated in the quiz, and their answers were roughly tabulated as follows: 20 percent of the physicians identified all four pictures correctly, as did 30 percent of the nurses, and 50 percent of the educators. The overall average was 30 percent.

Experimental work with animals shows a loss of secondary sexual characteristics after two or three generations on impoverished diets. Males lose their heavy masculine frame and their general contour begins to resemble the female. Females also tend to lose their distinguishing build, so that both sexes approach a state of physical neutrality. The male no longer has the strength of body that normally makes him the breadwinner and dominant personality. The female no longer has the pelvic capacity for easy childbearing.

Observation of our young people reveals that humans are subjected to the same food deficiencies as are seen in The Cat Study. Foods have been progressively depleted of nutritional substances since the roller flour mill was invented right after the Civil War. Canning, packaging, pasteurizing, and homogenizing—all contribute to hereditary breakdown.

Nutrition and Diet

Nutrition and *diet* are words with different meanings. *Nutrition* means the total of the metabolic processes supporting life, prenatal and postnatal.

45

In the broadest sense, human nutrition depends upon the adequacy of the progenitors, the quality of the food, the climate, the emotional makeup, and education, as well as upon the illnesses and stresses an individual sustains during his growing years. *Diet* refers to specific nutrients or foods eaten by an individual.

There is a trend in social thinking to advocate the equalization of the mass diet. Food provided in quantity by new agricultural technology is assumed to be of adequate nutritional quality. However, the long-term effects of synthetic chemicals in animal feeds, of hormones to stimulate growth, and of pesticides for sanitation have not been determined. That their use helps produce foods that are beautiful in appearance and free from pest damage cannot be disputed, but that these foods are nutritionally adequate can be. In a similar vein, we are assessing the effects of air and water pollution on human nutrition.

Now, what are some of the indications that the average human diet is deficient? Surface indices easily recognized by a large portion of our population are: thin, splitting, peeling nails due to disturbance in protein assimilation, especially lysine; thin skin due to lack of fat, or the reverse, thick skin, which cannot be picked up between the fingers due to lack of iodine or to excessive carbohydrate intake; and dry, brittle, lack-luster hair caused by too little unsaturated fatty acid. Moreover, a poorly nutritioned individual is apt to be irritable and unpredictable without cause. Exhaustion, in varying degrees, is a universal symptom of deficiency.

Less apparent indices of deficient nutrition relate to the development of the bones and ligaments as well as dentofacial structures. Following chapters will discuss deficiencies in osseous and dentofacial structures. Here, we will concentrate on ligaments and joints. Signs of poor ligaments due to deficient nutrition can be seen from infancy on. The signs are: hyperextensile elbow joints, hyperextensile shoulder joints, hyperextensile knee joints with lateral play, wrist bones that can be pulled apart, waddling roll to the hips, weak ankles, and dynamically and statically flat feet.

A trained medical examiner can readily pick up these conditions on physical examination. Later, X-rays reveal these problems more clearly. By the time the bones and cartilages of the joints are completely developed, malalignments become obvious.

The following two cases seen in our clinic give an overall view of the healthy maturing child and of the deficient maturing child. The outlines given are very broad, but they indicate a general pattern that is repeated over and over again.

The first case involves a young man born to a mother who has a relatively uneventful pregnancy. Much of her diet is home grown and she has excellent health and maintains normal activity throughout. The young man is born with good strong ligaments and has good osseous centers of compact bone. During his childhood, his food intake is nutritionally optimal, and he continues to develop good bones, strong muscles, and tight ligaments. Accordingly, his coordination is excellent. By six to nine months, he can hold his weight on a bar, and before a year, he can chin. His chest is broad, and his lungs have good air capacity. His endurance is good, and he is not prone to infections or to the usual chronic childhood illnesses. Moreover, he has quite a sunny disposition.

He does suffer a metabolic upset from measles at age 1, which leaves scars on his bones that take three years to heal, but there are no residual effects. On entering school, he rarely misses a day; he is a good student and participates willingly in sports and games. As the years pass, he becomes known for his athletic superiority and proves to be a champion in high school and in college. At every level of development, his coordination remains superior to others due to his excellent ligamentous and osseous development; in fact, his ligaments and joints mature slightly in advance of the average. The young man generally has a record of an all-around achiever with the social popularity and esteem that go with such a record.

The second case involves a young man born to a mother who is fraught with severe metabolic problems before and throughout her pregnancy. Her diet is deficient in raw and fresh factors and high in denatured protein and carbohydrate. The young man is born with weak ligaments and porous bones. Raised on a deficient diet, he passes through a series of metabolic upsets, starting with poor assimilation of his formula, and continuing with frequent colds, bouts of asthma, and numerous injuries due to poor coordination. His ligaments are weak and his joints hyperextend.

This boy shuns physical activity and has to be forced to participate in school sports by his teachers and coaches. He shows no particular interest in his school work and spends most of his time tinkering with hot rods. When he reaches his teens, his ligaments remain lax, his muscles weak, and his bones soft. He remains accident prone, but now with automobiles as well as with physical activities. In general, he is slow to mature, keeps a high soprano voice until he is 15, and has many social problems of maladjustment.

Our clinical experience demonstrates that it is perfectly possible for a child to improve his physical fitness, tighten his ligaments, strengthen his muscles, and harden his bones. It also demonstrates that, as a child's health and well-being improve, his activity level improves, and many academic and social "problems" begin to resolve. But before these improvements can occur, he must be placed on an optimal nutritional program.

Chapter Nine

BREAST FEEDING

"Milk, The Importance of Its Source," "Influence of Breast Feeding on Facial Development"

The superiority of human milk for human babies is natural. Human milk is rich in structural proteins, fats, hormones, enzymes, and vitamins essential for the optimum growth of the human brain as well as the body. Its exact formula remains a secret and has not been duplicated in the laboratory.

Alterations in the metabolism of a mother can quickly reflect in the health of her nursing infant. A deficient mother will have deficient milk, and when her diet is improved, the improvement will affect her milk. The alert physician caring for a nursing infant does not take the baby off the breast as soon as an incompatibility arises, but on the contrary, he immediately attempts to treat the mother knowing well that the nursing infant will give him information far sooner than the mother as to the correctness of his treatment. For example, an infant developing a mild eczematoid rash while on the breast merely requires a minor alteration in the mother's fatty acid intake. The alteration may react on the infant as early as the next day, sometimes the next feeding. Though the metabolites from a mother's milk may be imperfect and require correction if adequate lactation is to take place, the alternative sources of milk may have far greater imperfections.

Oscar Erf frequently cites an experiment in which groups of twin calves are fed the same milk. One twin suckles, the other drinks from a bucket. At the end of the year, the marked superiority of the suckled calves is recognized by the cattle judges evaluating them.

Professor Erf thought that the oxygen churned into the milk by the act of milking altered the chemical composition of the milk so that it was not as nutritious as milk that was squeezed from the teat directly into the calf's mouth, and there is little question that oxygen changes delicate nutritive substances in milk. Of equal or greater effect, however, are the changes brought about by the processes of pasteurizing, condensing, homogenizing, and reconstituting milk. Add to this the deficient, dry-feed dietary of most dairy cattle, and you will find that cow's milk is usually a poor second to mother's milk. An exception to this exists in the case of an untreated hypothyroid mother. A high-quality, raw cow's milk proves superior to her milk.

There is another advantage to breast feeding. The active exercise in nursing provides a growth stimulant to the muscles of the face, neck, chest, and spine. Some of the strongest muscles of the human body are the facial muscles used for chewing. As the bony structures of children are soft and pliable, when the facial muscles are exercised, they pull on the bony structure of the skull and increase its size. The action of nursing provides initial exercise to the face, which is not found in the action of sucking milk from a bottle.

The breast-fed infant is forced to work to extract milk. The infant pulls, pushes, kicks, pounds with his fists, plays hide-and-seek and exercises every muscle in his face and every muscle in his back. He juts his jaw forward and pulls it back, using his pterygoids, his masseters, his temporals, his linguals, and his nuchal muscles as he enjoys his meal. In his exercising, he develops his malar processes, which from a medical perspective means nasal passageways with good drainage and less susceptibility to infection, more symmetrical dental arches, and regular dentition.

What about the bottle-fed baby? A rubber nipple does not have the soft warmth, the life, that causes it to respond to the infant's tug. It is dead; and if it doesn't deliver milk, there is no by-play between infant and mother. It just won't give. Baby bawls, swallows air, and has the lifeless thing thrust into his mouth again and again until the blockage problem is discovered. When a red-hot pin opens the nipple, the milk flows; it rushes out and over and down baby's cheeks, and baby almost drowns, but he does get his feeding. He burps up some liquid and is put back in his crib—frustrated.

No play, no exercise in the feeding process, just another squaller with colic. He did use some muscles, but an entirely different group than the breast-fed baby. He usually is placed on his back, bottle propped just so to maximize the flow of gravity and all the infant need do is suck, suck, suck— and he may be a sucker all his life as a result. How about his face muscles? His neck muscles? His back muscles? He has hardly moved for fear the bottle might roll off and be lost. His hands, feet, and their connections, the trunk, arms, and legs, move helplessly in the air.

Comparative Facial Development Between
Nursed and Bottle-Fed Infants

In the following study of 327 patients of all ages, we analyzed the effect of nursing and bottle feeding on the facial development of the malar processes. We attempted to eliminate the external variables most apt to influence facial development: (1) heredity, (2) nutrition, and (3) exercise. To limit the influence of heredity in our study, we selected patients from the white race. To limit the influence of nutrition, we chose patients from a professional and business class who enjoyed a similar intake of the more sought-after foods. This left exercise as the major variable. There were minor variables to discount also. For instance, the quality of a nursing mother's milk varies in proportion to her health; further, mother's milk contains growth-stimulating steroids and phosphatases not contained in pasteurized formulas. Finally, the majority of those who came to the clinic as patients did so because of respiratory ailments, and so this study is based on a group suffering from poor facial development to a greater or lesser degree.

The masseter is the chief muscle of chewing, and its bony origin in the malar prominence of the zygoma is easy to measure. The masseter pulls and stimulates the malar prominence to grow downward and laterally. A large malar prominence is of value not only because it protects the eye and has aesthetic value, but because it is the foundation for a powerful bite. The distance from the most lateral part of the right malar prominence to the corresponding part of the left malar prominence is called the bimalar distance, and it measures lateral malar growth. Just above the zygomatic bones are the frontal bones, which come down laterally to the eyes. The distance from the right zygomaticofrontal suture is called the biorbital distance. The bones near the zygomaticofrontal suture serve chewing as the malar prominences do.

The bimalar and biorbital bony landmarks have almost no fat over them, which makes them easy to measure. The difference between the two areas is important because the masseter muscle attaches to the malar prominence, but no muscle attaches to the zygomaticofacial suture. Therefore, the biorbital distance is a control against which the growth of the bimalar distance can be measured as it is influenced by sucking, suckling, and chewing.

Figure 9.1 shows how to measure the biorbital distance with a caliper (in later studies we used X-rays for even greater accuracy). Figure 9.2 shows how to measure the bimalar distance.

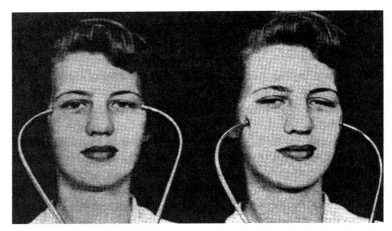

Fig. 9.1—Measuring the biorbital distance.   Fig. 9.2—Measuring the bimalar distance.

To determine the influence of nursing on facial development, the biorbital and bimalar distances of each individual are measured. The same physician made all the measurements and a nurse took a history of how long each patient had been nursed. Tables VIII and IX show our findings for the whole series.

Those individuals who are not nursed at all show the least malar growth. Those nursed three months or less show better malar growth, and those nursed more than three months show the best growth of all. In Table IX, we see that the percent of individuals who have well-developed malar processes depends on the length of time they are nursed as infants. Only 10.5 percent of those not nursed have a bimalar distance larger than their biorbital distance. Of those nursed three months or under, 23.6 percent have a bimalar distance larger than their biorbital distance. Breast feeding for more than three months causes the best facial development as 57.2 percent

TABLE VIII. CORRELATION OF NURSING AND MALAR GROWTH

LENGTH OF TIME NURSED	NUMBER OF CASES	BIORBITAL LARGER THAN BIMALAR	BIMALAR LARGER THAN BIORBITAL	BIORBITAL AND BIMALAR SAME SIZE
Not nursed	76	48	8	20
Nursed 3 months and under	55	34	13	8
Nursed more than 3 months	110	32	63	15
Nursed unknown length of time	86	11	61	14
Total number of cases	327	—	—	—

TABLE IX. CORRELATION OF NURSING AND MALAR GROWTH IN PERCENTAGES

LENGTH OF TIME NURSED	NUMBER OF CASES	BIORBITAL LARGER THAN BIMALAR	BIMALAR LARGER THAN BIORBITAL	BIORBITAL AND BIMALAR SAME SIZE
Not nursed	76	63.2%	10.5%	26.4%
Nursed 3 months and under	55	61.8%	23.6%	14.5%
Nursed more than 3 months	110	29.1%	57.2%	13.6%
Nursed unknown length of time	86	12.8%	71.0%	16.3%
Total number of cases	327	—	—	—

of these individuals have a bimalar distance greater than their biorbital distance.

In Tables X, XI, and XII, we analyze these patients by age groups. The following becomes apparent:

1. The malar processes grow at least until the age of 25.
2. The bimalar distance is less than the biorbital distance in most children under 12, regardless of the amount of nursing.
3. Nursing increases the percentage of children under 12 who have bimalar distances greater than biorbital distances.
4. After 12 years of age, more children have well-developed malar processes than have poorly developed ones. This is so only if they are nursed more than three months. If they are nursed for less than three months, the great majority have poorly developed zygomatic bones.
5. Most individuals over age 25 have fairly well-developed malar processes, regardless of whether or not they are nursed as infants, but good malar development is still more common among the ones who are well-nursed.

TABLE X. CORRELATION OF NURSING AND MALAR GROWTH
CASES UNDER 12 YEARS OF AGE

LENGTH OF TIME NURSED	NUMBER OF CASES	BIORBITAL LARGER THAN BIMALAR	BIMALAR LARGER THAN BIORBITAL	BIORBITAL AND BIMALAR SAME SIZE
Not nursed	46	36	1	9
Nursed 3 months and under	36	25	6	5
Nursed more than 3 months	22	14	4	4
Nursed unknown length of time	1	1	0	0
Total number of cases	105	—	—	—

**TABLE XI. CORRELATION OF NURSING AND MALAR GROWTH
CASES UNDER 12 YEARS OF AGE IN PERCENTAGES**

LENGTH OF TIME NURSED	NUMBER OF CASES	BIORBITAL LARGER THAN BIMALAR	BIMALAR LARGER THAN BIORBITAL	BIORBITAL AND BIMALAR SAME SIZE
Not nursed	46	78.3%	2.2%	19.5%
Nursed 3 months and under	36	69.5%	16.7%	13.9%
Nursed more than 3 months	22	63.6%	18.2%	18.2%
Nursed unknown length of time	1	100%	—	—
Total number of cases	105	—	—	—

**TABLE XII. CORRELATION OF NURSING AND MALAR GROWTH
CASES 12 TO 25 YEARS OF AGE**

LENGTH OF TIME NURSED	NUMBER OF CASES	BIORBITAL LARGER THAN BIMALAR	BIMALAR LARGER THAN BIORBITAL	BIORBITAL AND BIMALAR SAME SIZE
Not nursed	8	5	1	2
Nursed 3 months and under	12	9	2	1
Nursed more tha 3 months	13	5	6	2
Nursed unknown length of time	7	2	3	2
Total number of cases	40	—	—	—

Why is good facial development important in a young child? Consider the disorders that come from poor development. A face that is narrow in the frontal region has crowded sinuses and a narrow dental arch. Crowded sinuses lead to respiratory problems, and a narrow dental arch leads to impactions, displaced teeth, malocclusions, and agnathia. These defects interfere with good nutrition as the afflicted individual often prefers thoroughly cooked and macerated foods because they are easier to chew. But foods so prepared have lost important nutritive elements. For example, heating tomatoes in contact with air destroys their vitamin C content. Cooking meats well done to make them tender denatures the unsaturated lipids that the body needs to make hormones. A patient on such a diet will not ingest the proper building blocks to nourish his body. His resistance to infections will be low, and he may develop degenerative diseases. The first step in giving a person the right nutrition is to make him able to eat the right foods in sufficient quantity. This depends on the adequacy of his facial development, the strength of his muscles, and the shape of his masticating bones.

Dentofacial deformity requiring mechanical reconstruction by the use of braces, retainers, and bands is a widespread problem. There can be no doubt that modern dentofacial problems are encouraged, if not actually caused, by defective diets, by pathologic conditions of the nose and throat, and by general poor health. There also can be no doubt that the study we conducted on 327 patients reveals that the wholesale bottle feeding of our infant population is contributing to this problem.

Chapter Ten

EXPERIMENTAL AND CLINICAL EVIDENCE OF THE VALUE OF RAW MILK

"Clinical and Experimental Evidence of Growth Factors in Raw Milk," "Clinical Evidence of the Value of Raw Milk," "A Fresh Look at Milk"

To the bacteriologist, milk has been a source of much inquiry because of its great potential as a culture medium for all kinds of bacteria. Those who work with milk are familiar with the difficulty of sterilizing it. Each form of life has its own thermal death point. Some are high, some are low. They differ in different media. While the death point of a bacterium in a dry medium may be one temperature, in a colloidal medium like milk, it may be another, and in an aqueous solution, still another.

The destruction of bacteria in milk by heat processing is assumed to be essential in preventive medicine because of the findings of Pasteur. However, there are many good properties of milk that also are affected by heat processing because the entire physiochemical state of the milk is altered. Colloids are precipitated and mineral salts thrown out. Hormones, including thyroid, insulin, and adrenal steroids are affected as well as enzymes essential to efficient metabolism. Minerals are rendered less soluble. Antibodies giving infants immunity to disease are affected. Though the destruction of these substances in pasteurization may not produce death as hostile bacteria may, their deficiency in milk may impair the lifelong health of a child. This may be shown in poor skeletal development, lower resistance to disease, or in degenerative problems such as allergy and arthritis.

Health officials can no longer in good conscience ignore the possibility that pasteurization of milk may be menacing the proper growth and development of many more individuals than it is protecting. It is time to take a fresh look at milk and milk production, and at other methods of insuring its quality and safety.

Oscar Erf of Randleigh Farm

A fresh look at milk was given by a unique man of action, Oscar Erf of Randleigh Farm. Erf wanted to find out why the bones of his high-producing

Jersey cows were becoming soft and arthritic so that the animals had to be slaughtered. Collecting a group of scientists and ecologists of varying disciplines to aid him, he set out to gain a thorough understanding of the biological cycle of soil, plant, and animal life.

Erf and his collaborators wanted to produce the type of environment necessary for raising the finest cattle in order to produce the finest milk. These men were imbued with the idea that their efforts must start with the soil, to be certain it would supply the nutrients needed for growing the best pasture, corn, sprouts, and other feed for the dairy cattle. They tested their process in feed improvement and, thus, in soil improvement, by giving the resulting cow's milk to laboratory animals.

Their experiments with feeds ran the gamut of freezing, drying, curing, and adding chemicals to preserve the maximum amount of vital elements in the hay and other feeds needed for the winter months. They discovered the desirability of preserving the optimum amount of grass juice and fresh factors in the feed, just as we discovered in our cat and guinea pig experiments. Specifically, they sprouted corn during the winter to provide the freshness factor as well as vitamins and enzymes. They even used ultraviolet lamps to irradiate the cattle to give them a greater amount of short rays. Their single purpose was to study the effects of the various dietaries on the health of the cows and on the health of laboratory animals fed their milk.

Seeking to add to their cows' contentment, they employed the radio, the exercise wheel, and other innovations. They placed small amounts of nitrogen and carbon dioxide in their automatic milking system to prevent oxidation of the milk. Sanitation was given top priority, and bacteriological studies were continually made to assure the purity and safety of the milk.

Erf's concept of quality control has given way to the concept of quantity production in our American society. Health experts spend their time trying to explain that one bottle of milk is just as good as another; that the meat from one steer, though it may taste different, has identical food value to that of another. At the same time, it is common to hear milk attacked as a cause of many human ailments, such as high cholesterol, arteriosclerosis, pyorrhea, and allergy. It must be asked: "Is it possible that a food that has nurtured man since the earliest agrarian times has suddenly become harmful to him?"

Erf's answer to this question is very simple: When the nutrition of cows is poor, the nutritional value of their milk is poor. Through his research, he was convinced that milk can only be as health-giving as the health of the cow producing it; consequently, when cow's milk is deficient in trace elements important for proper metabolism, faulty metabolism will occur in the consumer—animal or man. Erf considered that imposed faulty metabolism is the cause of deficiency problems and proposed that an allergic cow produces an allergic human being.

High Cholesterol and Other Problems

To the specific charges that milk causes high cholesterol, pyorrhea, arthritis, and allergies, our own research suggests the following answers:

Cholesterol: The specific charge that milk produces high cholesterol in humans is largely based on the premise that the ingestion of cholesterol and the deposit of cholesterol are the same. The biochemist, using tracer elements, has been unable to show that the ingestion of cholesterol will elevate cholesterol in the body. Extensive use of quality raw milk, cream, and farm eggs with tuberculous patients at the sanatorium failed to produce a single case of hypercholesterolemia and atheroma. A lifetime consumption of clean, fresh, raw milk from healthy cattle does not produce metabolic disease in man. Cholesterol is not the villain; the villain is what man does to his cattle and milk.

Pyorrhea and Arthritis: Experiments initiated by Erf show that pasteurized milk produces pyorrhea in cats and imperfect development of rat incisors. Our own research on cats shows that poor quality and heat-processed milks cause osteoporosis and certain types of arthritis in cats and rats. Such deficiency diseases can be traced back to deficiencies of fresh, vital elements found in raw foods in the dietary.

Allergies: As indicated by Erf, methods of processing and preserving foods enter into the problem of digestion and immunity. The digestive mechanisms, both enteral and cellular, permit infants, children, and adults to become sensitive when elements controlling the permeability of cells are altered. The heat processing of foods destroys elements that protect us from digestive and immunological problems. Some individuals who become sensitized to subquality milk can never be desensitized, and milk should be removed from their diet. This does not mean that milk should be downgraded as a nonessential food. Optimum raw milk is one of the best and cheapest foods available for infants and children. Emphasis should return to improving the quality of the milk produced so that it won't be lacking in the essential substances that insure proper assimilation and protect against allergy.

The ideas that animals producing food for man should be healthy in their domesticated environment and that this imposed environment should be designed to provide optimum health for man are lost. In our fear of meeting hard challenges successfully, we are burying our heads in the sand and ignoring the fact that our modern methods of production may be rendering valuable foods dangerous. We cannot afford to pasteurize milk if it is found that pasteurization diminishes the potency of the growth-promoting factors that determine the skeletal development of our children. We cannot afford to lessen the resistance of our children to respiratory infection, asthma, bronchitis, and the common cold. Essential minerals, fats, proteins, hormones, enzymes, and antibodies—all present in the finest raw milk—promote good health among young and old alike. If we are to practice true preventive medicine and optimize the health of the human race, we must take the necessary steps not only to insure the safety of the milk, but to insure its nutritional value.

Chapter Eleven

MILK AND THE HUMAN SKELETON

"The Clinical Significance of the Osseous System," "Clinical Evidence of the Value of Raw Milk," "Deficient Calcification Produced by Diet: Experimental and Clinical Considerations"

Webster's International Dictionary defines the *skeleton* as "the bones of a human being or other vertebrate collectively; the bony or more or less cartilaginous framework supporting the soft tissues and protecting the internal organs." Yet, the skeleton is much more than this. It is a mineral storehouse as well as a blood-building organ. The fluidity of the skeleton's mineral content and its relationship to the electrolytic, hence physiologic balance, is critical to the health of the individual. The bones are living organs, which not only act as supportive tissues for the muscles and organs, but also as dynamic units whose biological efficiency must be in proportion to the functional activity of the body as a whole. The size of the skeleton as compared to the size of the body, the density of the bones, and the appearance and time of closure of the epiphyses provide evidence of the efficiency of the individual's growth and development.

One of our specific measurements for comparing and evaluating the quality of children's nutrition is the density of their bones as revealed by X-ray. We use the density of bones as an index of the amount of minerals available for physiological processes. The child, who has a compact cortex and compact trabeculation, has a much higher electrolytic reserve than the child who has the same size bones with a relatively coarse mesh. Moreover, when the size of the shaft of the bone is considered in relation to its mineral density, we can project a child's muscular development into adulthood. For instance, it is impossible for a fine-boned skeleton to support the musculature necessary for hard physical labor, just as it is impossible for a child with a small body frame to become a professional football player.

Lack of bone mineralization is playing an ever-increasing role among the aged, causing spontaneous crushing of vertebrae, particularly those of the lower thoracic and lumbar regions. The softness of these spinal bones and their inability to bear body weight are causing many old people to spend their last years in misery. Fractures of the neck of the femur among the elderly are precipitating more deaths than in the past, and we are seeing an increasing number of these fractures in the middle aged. Even the young are suffering more bone fractures as a result of trivial accidents in their gymnasiums or on their playgrounds.

Deficient Calcification

A normal supply of calcium and its proper utilization are important to an individual throughout life. Evidence is developing that calcium deficiency is not uncommon. Even though the ordinary diet is supposed to be adequate in its calcium content, it is only necessary to look at the teeth, facial development, and osseous problems of all ages to recognize that something is wrong with the calcium metabolism of a large percentage of our population. In order to influence calcification in patients, we have given them diets rich in calcium, have administered quantities of calcium salts over long periods of time, and have administered vitamins to aid assimilation, and yet we have been unable to establish normal calcium utilization.

This failure suggests that some factor or factors are lacking in the ordinary diet, which are necessary for the proper assimilation and deposition of this mineral in the bones. Ruling out a lack of exposure to the mineral itself, we began correlating our clinical findings with our findings in The Cat Study. Cats on fresh, raw foods have no apparent problems utilizing the calcium in their diet and have strong bones, but the cats on cooked foods suffer symptoms of calcium deficiency not unlike those of our patients. By adding fresh and raw foods to our patients' diets, a marked improvement became noticeable in their calcium assimilation as recorded in their X-rays. Again, it suggests that heat labile substances in foods exert control over calcium utilization in cats and humans alike, and that these substances are destroyed by heat and oxidation.

Effects of Different Milks on Bone Development

The following study of 150 children drinking different types of milk compares their bone age and skeletal structures. The bone-age tables of

Engelbach (22) are used. We make a somewhat arbitrary adjustment to the standard we use for normal because, if we use the bones of a breast-fed, hardy farm boy or girl as the standard for normal, 95 percent of the children in our study would show deficiency. By adjusting our normal standard, only 54 percent reveal deficiency. Our classification of "poorly calcified" is also somewhat arbitrarily based on our X-ray studies of the calcification of the bones in the wrist, feet, and tip of the clavicle.

There are 31 infants in this study who are breast fed for six months or more. Among these, nineteen show maternal histories of thyroid dys-function, and others have histories of severe genital disorders. Bearing in mind that the activity of the thyroid is closely associated with the develop-ment of the skeleton and that the deficiencies of the mother are apparently transferred to the offspring, it is not surprising that many of these 31 in-fants present deficiencies. On the basis of the Engelbach studies, eighteen of the children show delay in the development of the centers of ossifica-tion, four are slightly advanced, and nine are normal. Seven children have fine bones, and seven show large, poorly calcified bones with weak joints of the rachitic type.

Six children in the study receive raw certified milk, five taking the milk without modification. In this group, the osseous and skeletal developments are excellent. Four drink metabolized vitamin D milk and, of these, two show a slight advance in the osseous development, one is normal, and one shows delay.

Another group of eight children on raw milk formulas shows no deviation from standard in their osseous centers. One shows a fine bone development.

The largest single group in this study consists of 43 children fed canned milk. The so-called adapted milks (prepared formulas such as Similac) are not segregated from the milk powders or from the condensed milks because we find little if any difference in their effects on ossification. The striking features of this group of 43 children is that over one-half (23) have very fine, small bones; nine have marked disturbances in calcification, though the bones are of normal size or larger than normal, and nine exhibit marked weaknesses in their joints and ligaments. When the bone age of all the children is calculated, 23 are below the normal standard for their age, fifteen are normal, and five are above normal.

When ten babies fed pasteurized milk formula are studied, four are de-layed in ossification, three are normal, and three are advanced beyond their age. The bones of seven are fine, one is normal, and two are rachitic.

In another group of 34 children given boiled milk formula, 21 show delayed bone age, twelve are normal, and one is advanced. Eighteen have fine osseous development, six show normal development, and ten are of the poorly calcified, large bone class.

Two children on formula containing no milk or milk products show delayed bone age with enlarged, weak joints.

Comparative X-Ray Studies

Figure 11.1 A represents an X-ray of a nine-month-old boy nursed nine months by a healthy mother eating a diet rich in fresh foods grown on her own farm. The baby has bones of large diameter. His development is normal for his age, and he has fully recovered from the period of lowered calcification that follows birth. His skull is large, he has a well-developed dental arch, and has ample space for all his teeth. His soft tissues are of excellent tone, and X-rays suggest excellent calcification.

Figure 11.1 B represents an infant of similar age to A. The mother is hypothyroid and unable to nurse her child. The baby is placed on undiluted raw cow's milk of the best grade obtainable. He has smaller bones, not quite as dense as those of A, but of fair quality. He shows a fair recovery from the normal lowered calcification following birth, has good facial development, but inferior to that of A. Bones from X-ray studies suggest good calcification, but again less than A. Tissue tone is good.

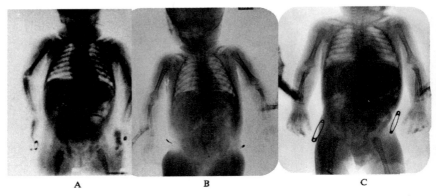

Fig. 11.1—X-ray of 3 nine-month-old infants. A, Healthy infant nursed by healthy mother. B, Caesarian infant born of hypothyroid mother, given raw cow's milk formula. C, deficient infant from deficient mother; given cooked milk formulas.

64

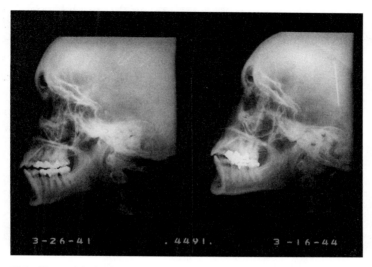

Fig. 11-2—X-ray of skull of female, age 38. Developed fully on good diet until age of 19, then on deficient diets for nineteen years.

Figure 11.1 C shows the skeleton of an infant whose mother has many symptoms of deficiency. She is unable to nurse her child. The baby is placed on all kinds of cooked milk formulas. As a result, he makes a poor recovery from the lowered calcification following birth. He shows delay in osseous development, has small bones, distorted facial structures, and is generally deficient in physiologic reaction.

Figure 11-2 shows the skull of a well-developed female, age 38, whose good diet carries her through her growing years until at 19, she decides it is necessary to economize on her food in order to "succeed" in her chosen work. She loses her third molars and develops cavities in four more teeth. Some of her bones are slightly more radio translucent than normal. However, though suffering from a prolonged period of starvation, she still has a fundamentally excellent body. Her height is 5 feet 3 inches, and she has large bones, a broad thorax, a large body, and short legs. The upper and lower halves of her body are of equal length.

Figure 11.3 represents the skull of an individual who belongs to the third generation of individuals on deficient diets. The family history of deficiency includes the mother and grandmother. Her age is the same as that of Figure 11.2, 38 years. She is 6 feet tall, and her bony structures show

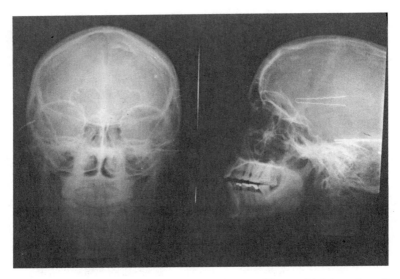

Fig. 11.3—Skull of female, age 38. Deficient development. History of deficiency in mother and grandmother.

poor calcification. She has a poorly developed skull and has small bones, a small thorax, and has lost most of her teeth. The lower half of her body is much longer than the upper half. She lacks the vitality to work more than one day a week.

The pattern of calcification of a child depends upon the diet and health of the mother; and in the case of Figure 11.3, on the grandmother and perhaps remoter ancestors as well. The pattern of calcification also depends on whether or not the infant is nursed, and if not nursed, on what type of formula it is raised. Our experimental work proves that an adequate amount of heat labile substances are necessary in a mother's milk, as well as in any substitute food, in order for proper calcification of the skeleton to take place. It is these very substances that are destroyed in pasteurized and boiled milk formulas and in the cooked foods later added to a child's diet.

In applying what we have learned in The Cat Study and in our clinical experience, we find that there is little that can be done to change the calcification that is established at the end of a child's growing period. If a child's calcification is poor at this time, it will remain poor throughout his life. On the positive side, it is possible to improve the calcification of children who are still growing and have been on deficient diets by giving them the highest grade of raw milk, raw meat, raw vegetables, and fresh fruits.

Chapter Twelve

THE EFFECT OF DISTURBED NUTRITION
ON BONES DEVELOPING UNDER STRESS

"Studies of Fragmentation of the Tarsal and Metatarsal Bones Resulting from Recurrent Metabolic Insults," "The Effect of Disturbed Nutrition on Dentofacial Structures," "Fragmentation and Scarring of the Tarsal and Metatarsal Bones," "Nutritional Aspects of the Orthodontic Problem," "The Effect of Diet on the Nutrition of the Dental Patient"

Prenatal Disturbances

Though all organs of the body are integrated in the developmental process, they form *in utero* according to a staggered time schedule. Consider the dentofacial structures alone. The mandibular arch in the fetus begins to develop about the twenty-eighth day, and the dental ridge begins to develop between the fortieth and forty-fifth day. The germs of the deciduous teeth form about the sixty-fifth day, and the first permanent molar bud is formed by the fourth month. Calcification of the enamel organ begins during the fifth month. A series of X-ray studies reveal that metabolic disturbances of the mother during pregnancy can affect the adequacy of the oral structures of the infant.

In a group of fifteen children with very small deciduous teeth and narrow arches, histories of serious metabolic disturbance and accompanying dietary insufficiencies occur in the first three months of pregnancy. For example, serious nutritional disturbances during the seventh week of pregnancy correlate with the receding mandible and developmental failure of the maxillary portion of the face (Figure 12.2) and in the protruding mandible (Figure 12.1).

The influence of the dietary on the anterior portion of the face is dramatic. During the pregnancy of the older child, the mother suffers extreme emotional tension with accompanying malnutrition. This child shows a narrow and poorly developed face. She has very small primary dentition and the inferior development of her mandible and maxilla is reflected in the paranasal sinuses and structures beneath the base of her brain.

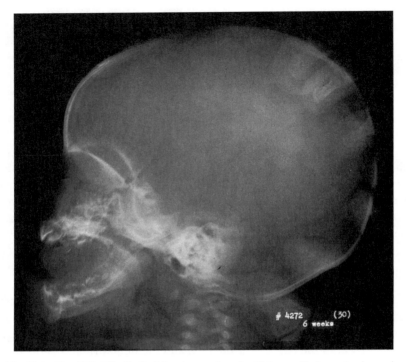

Fig. 12.1—No. 4272 (30). Skull of female, age 6 weeks. Note mandibular protrusion and small middle third of face.

During the pregnancy of the younger child, the mother enjoys relatively good physical and emotional health and eats an optimum diet. In addition, this child is given a superior nutritional program to that of her sister at the same age and never suffers the recurrent metabolic upsets of her sister. It is evident that this girl has developed a regular mandible and adequate room in the anterior portion of the mouth for all of her teeth, and that her mandible is larger than that of her sister who is two years older. Likewise, its length is greater and the thickness of the rami is heavier. Her coronoid processes show superior muscular development. The younger child shows breadth of oral structures and symmetry of face in contrast to her sister whose nares are pinched and whose nasal passageways are so small that her tonsils and adenoids are a problem.

Postnatal Disturbances

After an infant is born, dietary deficiencies leave their mark on the bones, developing under the stresses of chewing and walking. Routine

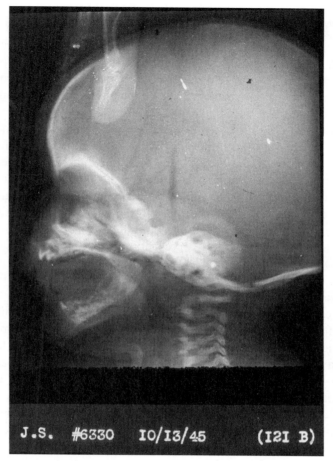

J.S. #6330 IO/I3/45 (I2I B)

Fig. 12.2—No. 6330. Eleven-day-old female infant. Receding mandible. Mother suffered extreme anemia and was very ill throughout pregnancy.

X-rays are taken of the lateral and anterioposterior views of the skull, of the hands, and of the feet. Particular attention is given to the bones of the feet of children between the ages of 3 months and 6 years as they learn to walk. (Figures 12.5, 12.6, and 12.7)

The first evidence of fragmentation of the bones is in the internal structures of the talus, cuboid, or calcaneium and appears as quickly as the third month (Figure 12.5). Obvious fragmentation does not begin, as a rule, until the child starts to use his feet in walking. By the second year, the cuboid, navicular, and three cuneiform bones may be severely involved. Fragmentation of the bases of metatarsals two, three, four, and five and the proximal epiphysis of the metatarsal of the first digit may be noted

71

(Figure 12.6). In many children there is a disturbance in the proximal epiphysis of the first phalanx. As the epiphyseal heads of the metatarsal bones develop, they may not appear in a regular order, but frequently as semiheads or fragmented heads, or they may appear at a much later time than is normally expected. This fragmentation reaches its maximum severity between the third and fourth years.

In X-rays of children taken at six-month intervals, we see the process of healing begin at the bases of the metatarsals between the fourth and fifth years (Figure 12.7). At the same time, the cuneiform bones and the navicular bone are beginning to become smooth. The third cuneiform usually shows signs of healing first. By the time the child is six years old, the epiphyseal heads are largely healed, but the navicular bone and the first cuneiform may still show signs of some unhealed fragmentation. Occasionally, active fragmentation is present up to and including the seventh year. The scars formed during the healing process are formed by a thickening of internal condensation of the trabeculae in the internal structure of the bone.

Between the tenth and eleventh years, when the epiphysis of the base of the fifth metatarsal appears, new evidence of fragmentation may occur.

During the period of marked fragmentation of the bones of the feet, a child may show little or no outward evidence of extensive bone damage. He may limp for a brief period, or his foot may become flat. He rarely complains of pain. Yet, it is entirely possible that the widespread prevalence of tarsal and metatarsal failure in the deficient child may account for the crippling foot disturbances of later life and may be the forerunner of arthritis.

In Figure 12.8, a boy patient experiences profound difficulty in becoming established on an agreeable nutritional program. His mother suffers from severe anemia during her pregnancy and is unable to nurse him. By the age of three months, this boy develops chronic bronchitis and asthma, which is paralleled by visible disturbances in the osseous development. The bones of his feet are particularly affected. Healing of the basal epiphysis is not complete at three years, ten months (Figure 12.9), and requires another year to appear normal (Figure 12.10).

The quality of the diet, prenatal and postnatal, affects the osseous structures. Though the foot is the easiest of the structures of the lower extremities to study, the ankle, the knee, and the hip may show disturbances in growth equally as well. The carpals and the metacarpals of the hand are not under as severe stress at the same developmental time as the corresponding

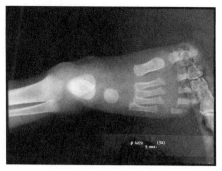

Fig. 12.5—No. 4272 (32). Foot of female, age 3 months. Marked angulation and concavity of the distal end of metatarsals 2, 3, 4, and 5. Slight condensation of the internal trabecular structure of the cuboid.

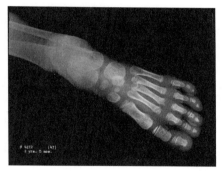

Fig. 12.6—No. 4272 (47). Foot of female, age 2 years, 5 months. Slight fragmentation of cuneiform 1 and 3. Mild roughness of navicular. Some roughness and fragmentation of bases of metatarsals 2, 3, 4, and 5. No epiphyseal head of metatarsal 5. Metatarsal 4 shows epiphyseal head just appearing. Three is fragmented. Two is poorly developed. Proximal epiphysis of metatarsal 1 is rough.

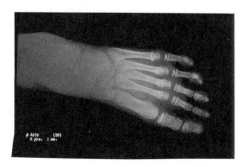

Fig. 12.7—No. 4272 (59). Foot of female, age 5 years, 1 month. Largely healed. Slight condensation at base of metatarsals. A little roughness of cuneiform 1.

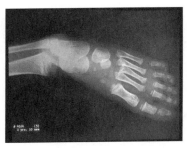

Fig. 12.8—No. 4164 (3). Foot of male, age 2 years, 10 months. Child suffered many recurrent metabolic upsets in form of asthmatic attacks. Note fragmentation of the bases of metatarsals. Increased fragmentation of proximal heads of metatarsal 1. Evidence of disturbance in mesial distal head of metatarsal 1; beginning fragmentation at head of metatarsal 1. Failure of heads to develop on metatarsals 3, 4, and 5. Cuneiform 1 fragmented. Cuneiform 2 fragmented. Cuneiform 3 rough and fragmented. Some internal condensation.

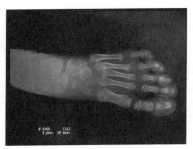

Fig. 12.9—No. 4164 (11). Foot of male, age 3 years, 10 months. Metatarsal 5 shows continued healing of the base. Healing just begun in metatarsal 4. Base of metatarsals 2 and 3 still clearly fragmented. Metatarsal head of 2 beginning to develop. Metatarsal 3 bifid, 4 and 5 still delayed. Frank osteochondrosis noted at the head of metatarsal 1, and proximal epiphysis still fragmented. Navicular and cuneiforms 1 and 2 still fragmented. Cuneiform 3 largely healed.

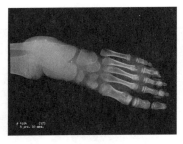

Fig. 12.10—No. 4164 (17). Foot of male, age 4 years, 10 months. Bases of 4 and 5 essentially healed. Note internal condensation in bases. Two and 3 still healing with internal condensation evident. Proximal epiphysis of 1 largely healed. Distal portion of 1 shows osteochondritis still present. Epiphysis of 2 fairly well developed, 3 still bifid. Four came in as hemiepiphysis. Five not yet present. Second cuneiform almost healed. Navicular and first cuneiform healing. Internal condensation in all distal bones.

bones of the foot. The child does not begin to use his hand for heavy work until after the sixth year. By this time, the formation of the carpal bones is well along, and the epiphyseal heads and the bases of the meta-carpals are thoroughly developed. Therefore, no definite correlation can be drawn between the hand and foot, with the possible exception that the carpal bones may show a suggestive concomitant fragmentation of the internal trabeculation. Figures 12. 11 and 12.12 show the foot and hand for comparison.

Correlations can be made between the fragmentation found in the foot and malformation of the dentofacial structures (Figures 12.13 and 12.14).

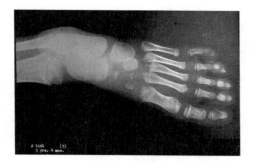

Fig. 12.11—No. 4164 (7). Foot of male, age 3 years, 4 months. Note extensive fragmentation of the metatarsal bases continuing, with slight amount of healing of metatarsal 5. Continued fragmentation of metatarsals 2, 3, and 4. Appearance of metatarsal heads is still delayed. Proximal epiphysis of metatarsal 1, still fragmented. Metatarsal head of 1 shows increased condensation. Internal condensation noted in cuboid and third cuneiform. Fragmentation of cuneiforms 1 and 2, and navicular, still prominent.

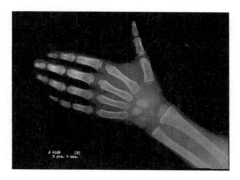

Fig. 12.12—No. 4164 (8). Hand of male, age 3 years, 4 months. The capitate and hamate still show internal condensation and coarse internal trabeculation of the bones. Otherwise essentially normal.

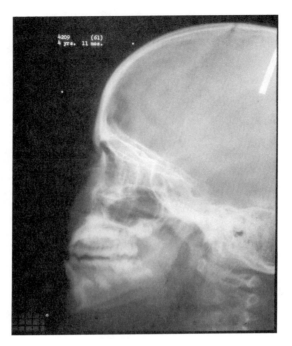

Fig. 12.13—No. 4209 (61). Skull of female, age 4 years, 11 months. Failure in forward movement of middle third of the face and base of skull, giving an apparent mandibular protrusion.

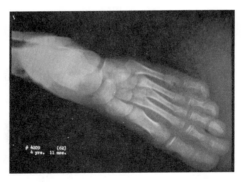

Fig. 12.14—No. 4209 (62). Foot of female, age 4 years, 11 months. Notice internal condensation in base of metatarsals, third cuneiform, navicular, and cuboid. Third cuneiform is apparently not quite healed.

The time between three months and six years corresponds to the erupting and early shedding of deciduous teeth, to the expanding of the dental arches to make room for permanent dentition, and to the budding of the

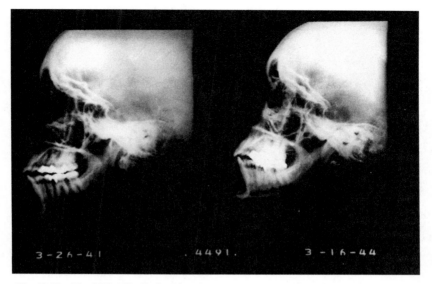

Fig. 12.15—No. 4491 (47). Skull of female, age 32 years, before improvement in dietary (left), and three years later (right), after giving birth to two children. Note changes in skull configuration and laying down of scar bone.

permanent teeth, except for the third molars. It also corresponds to the formation of the metatarsal bones and of the epiphyses and to the completion and articulation of the metatarsal bones with the cuboid and cuneiform bones and with each other. Whenever deficiency in the osseous structure and coarse trabeculation of the jawbone can be seen, severe metatarsal fragmentation in the foot can also be seen.

The scars which are laid down in the bones during periods of fragmentation appear to be permanent. Adult patients, who have dentofacial failures, show scars in the bones of their feet similar to those found in children. Though it appears impossible to remove the scars themselves and impossible to change the developmental patterns of bones, it is possible to improve organ efficiency and to alter structural development. As mentioned, it is possible for an adult to rebuild calcium in his bones by consuming adequate quantities of growth-promoting substances found in fresh and raw foods. The new bone laid down in regeneration is not the original bone repaired, but is a scar bone (Figure 12.15).

X-rays and photographs (Figures 12.16, 12.17, 12.18, and 12.19) show the recovery of a five-year-old girl with a disfiguring mandibular protrusion. Placed on a diet rich in growth and developmental activators, and

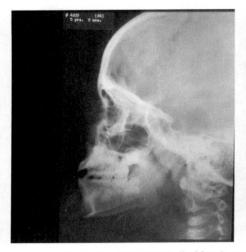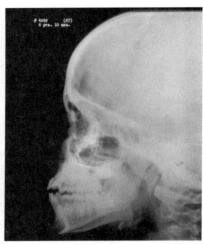

Fig. 12.16—No. 4209 (64). Skull of female, age 5 years, 9 months. Middle third and base of skull showing forward movement..

Fig. 12.17—No. 4209 (67). Skull of female, age 6 years, 10 months. Further progress.

encouraged to use her facial structures by chewing tough objects and by making faces, the girl shows remarkable improvement by the age of ten. Though no orthodontic treatment is applied, her mandibular protrusion is largely corrected by the development of the middle third of her face. This child is representative of a group of children who experience improvement in facial development solely because of dietary improvement (Figures 12.20 and 12.21).

Improvement of the facial configuration of deficient children can be either progressive or retrogressive. We have had the opportunity of noting broadening and development of the middle face by applying the principles learned from our research on cats. We have had the sad experience of seeing children, who materially improve during a two-to-three-year period, show a definite retrogression because they suddenly decide that the details of their dietary program are too irksome for them to continue. It is logical to assume that children who have fundamental structural weaknesses will lose what they gain more easily when they revert to a poor diet.

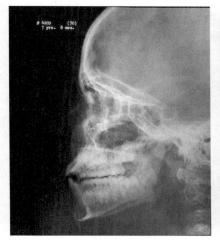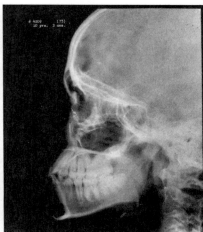

Fig. 12.18—No. 4209 (70). Skull of female, age 7 years, 8 months. Malar prominence moving forward. Glabellar prominence beginning to develop.

Fig. 12.19—No. 4209 (73). Skull of female, age 10 years, 2 months. Notice changing angle of upper teeth. Good alignment of teeth. Good forward projection of face and base of brain case. Series shows increase in growth of middle portion of face in respect to mandible.

Nutritional Principles

In applying the principles learned from our experimental work with cats to human beings, we find that (1) all people are influenced by preceding generations and (2) people can be healthy only if the stock from which they come is healthy, and the food they eat is adequate.

Since the individual is a product of heredity, both germ-plasm and chemical, the way he develops after birth depends on the nutrition of his inheritance as well as on his own nutrition. For this reason, nutrition becomes one of the most important elements in preventive medicine. Good food is important to the infant, the adolescent, the adult, and especially to the expectant mother. At any age, injury can be done by an inadequate diet. Inadequacy in infancy and childhood alters development; in later life, it affects the efficiency of organic function, reproductivity, and general physiologic activity.

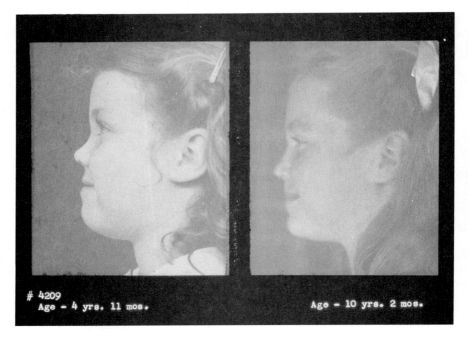

Fig. 12.20—No. 4209. Lateral views of patient at 4 years, 11 months of age, and 10 years, 2 months of age, showing changes in facial configuration and tissue stability.

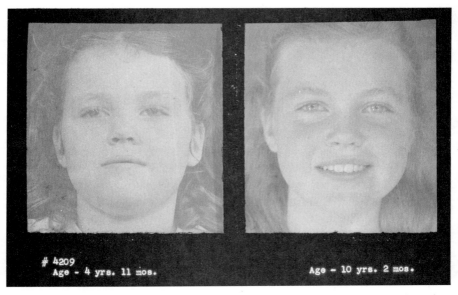

Fig. 12.21—No. 4209. Frontal view of patient at 4 years, 11 months of age and 10 years, 2 months of age.

Scientists first thought they had established that good nutrition depends upon the adequate intake of proteins, carbohydrates, fats, and minerals only to realize later that hormones, enzymes, and vitamins are just as essential to the building and maintenance of the human body. They are just beginning to realize that these vital growth substances are destroyed by modern methods of milling, heating, and processing foods; and moreover, that modern methods of agriculture and animal husbandry are depleting the soil and depleting the quality of plant and animal products that furnish these substances to our diet.*

We cannot go back and change the ancestors of our children, but we can prescribe a diet that is adequate not only from the standpoint of proteins, fats, carbohydrates, and minerals, but from the standpoint of hormones, enzymes, and vitamins.

---

*Ed. This is still true. The progress made since this was written has been at best glacial.

Part Three

Chapter Thirteen

RECIPROCAL RELATIONSHIP OF THE HEALTH
OF PLANTS, ANIMALS, AND HUMAN BEINGS

"Reciprocal Relationship of the Health of Plants, Animals and Human Beings,"
*"The Effect of Heat-Processed Foods and Metabolized Vitamin D Milk on the
Dentofacial Structures of Experimental Animals"*

Man is part of a biological cycle. The continued development of optimum human beings requires that this cycle be maintained. The soil is the first element in this cycle and is vitalized by the bacteria that inhabit it. The bacteria provide food for the earthworms, which process the soil through their bodies, converting organic matter into humus, and humus provides food for the growth of plants, supporting animal and human life. When the excreta of animals and humans is returned to the soil, it nourishes the bacteria and so allows the biological cycle to go on ad infinitum.

That healthy plants are essential to animal life and that animal excrement acts as a soil rejuvenator is widely recognized, but that possible harm is done to human life when disturbances or deficiencies occur in any phase of the biological cycle is not widely recognized.

Modern man has gleaned his fields to fill his larder, but his system of sanitary engineering has destroyed most of the soil-rejuvenating, organic materials. No longer does man return to the soil those materials taken from the soil. Instead he pours them into the ocean and loses them to his civilization. Harsh mineral fertilizers, which destroy soil bacteria and earthworms, are being substituted for the organic compost of the past to the long-range detriment of the soil at one end of the biological cycle and of human life at the other.

A chance observation led us to experiment with the growth properties of the excreta in the pens of the cats on various cooked and raw diets. As feeding experiments are completed, pens become empty. Shortly, weeds sprout in them, but with noticeable differences in their size and health. As

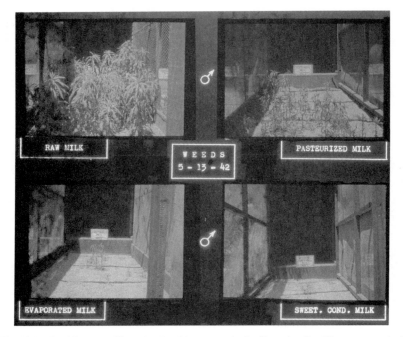

Fig. 13.1—Pen 18—raw milk, males. Pen 20—pasteurized milk, males. Pen 22—evaporated milk, males. Pen 24—sweetened condensed milk, males.

can be seen in Figures 13.1, 13.2, 13.3, and 13.4, the number of weeds in the pens and their hardiness appears to be in direct relationship to the health and vigor of the animals that lived in them. Planting navy beans in the pens, we find that the same growth patterns result. See Table XIII.

We ran a controlled experiment in 1939 to confirm these findings and another controlled experiment in 1940 to see if there would be any difference in the fertilizing values of composted manure from healthy and unhealthy cats.

Navy Bean Experiment—1939

In this initial experiment, navy beans are planted in three different plots. The first plot is fertilized with noncomposted excreta of cats fed raw meat. The second plot is fertilized with noncomposted excreta of cats fed cooked meat, and the third plot is not fertilized. When the first crop of navy beans is harvested from the three plots, the beans show no apparent difference in their size, color, or shape. However, when they are planted

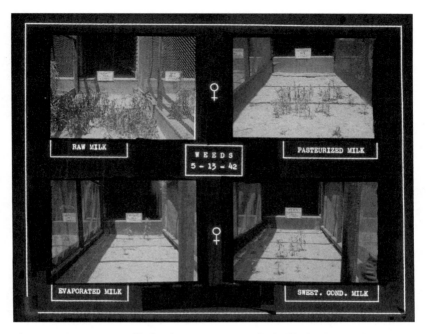

Fig. 13.2— Pen 17—raw milk, females. Pen 19—pasteurized milk, females. Pen 21—evaporated milk, females. Pen 23—sweetened condensed milk, females.

to produce a second generation, their germination rates differ. The plot fertilized with raw meat shows 88 percent germination, the plot fertilized with cooked meat shows 72 percent germination, and the unfertilized plot shows 96 percent germination.

Two weeks after planting, the unfertilized plants are the tallest, and the plants fertilized with raw meat and cooked meat are about equal in height. The plants fertilized with raw meat have the best form and color.

Three weeks after planting, the group of plants fertilized with cooked meat is the tallest, the unfertilized group the next tallest, and the group fertilized with raw meat is the shortest. This rate of growth is exhibited throughout the experiment. The plants fertilized with cooked meat are pale green in color, have many more stems and leaves, and their stalks are thinner than the plants of the other two groups. Plants fertilized with raw meat are short and squat, have much deeper color, and are sturdier than the plants fertilized with cooked meat. The unfertilized plants are intermediate between the groups fertilized with raw and cooked meat with respect to the above features. The leaves of the plants fertilized with cooked meat are

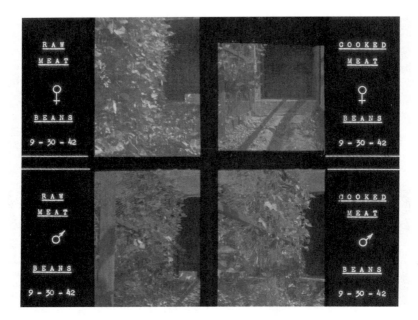

Fig. 13.3—Pen 13—cooked meat, females. Pen 14—cooked meat, males. Pen 15—raw meat, males. Pen 16—raw meat, females.s

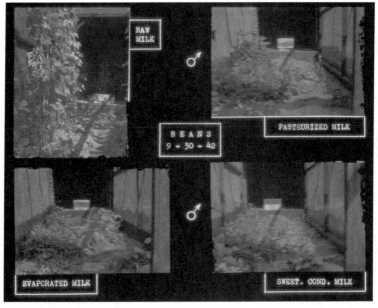

Fig. 13.4—Pen 18—raw milk, males. Pen 20—pasteurized milk, males. Pen 22—evaporated milk, males. Pen 24—sweetened condensed milk, males.

TABLE XIII. NAVY BEANS PLANTED IN PENS OF EXPERIMENTAL CATS

	PEN	COLOR	GROWTH	FIRST BLOSSOMS	NO. OF BLOSSOMS	PERIOD OF BLOOM	NO. OF BEANS	NO. OF PODS	BEANS PER POD	LIFE OF PLANT (DAYS)
Cooked meat-0 Males & Females	13	good slightly yellow	mixed poor & excellent	70 days	500	49 days	700	134	5.2	147
Cooked meat-# Males & Females	14	good slightly yellow	mixed poor & excellent	63 days	2500	49 days	1886	451	4.2	147
Raw meat Males	15	deep green	extra-thick stems	77 days	2000	70 days	1142	357	3.2	161
Raw meat Females	16	deep green	excellent	91 days	1800	56 days	684	220	3.1	161
Raw milk Females	17	bright green	good	63 days	550	49 days	1092	328	3.3	126
Raw milk Males	18	bright green	good	63 days	1200	49 days	3487	659	5.3	147
Pasteurized milk Females	19	poor	weak	63 days	500	42 days	615	146	4.2	126
Pasteurized milk Males	20	fair	fair	63 days	600	35 days	1045	298	3.5	126
Evaporated milk Females	21	fair	weak fine stems	63 days	300	49 days	120	42	2.8	126
Evaporated milk Males	22	fair	weak sprawled	63 days	300	49 days	339	126	2.7	126
Sweetened Condensed milk Females	23	fair	poor	63 days	350	49 days	190	69	2.7	112
Sweetened Condensed milk Males	24	fair	poor weak stems	63 days	350*	42 days	1252	407*	3.0	119

* Counts were made weekly. Some blossoms were probably missed.
-0 Breeding pen normally housed female cats.
-# Breeding pen normally housed male cats.

TABLE XIV. ANALYSIS OF NAVY BEANS: FIRST GENERATION

TYPE OF FERTILIZER USED ON NAVY BEANS	MOISTURE (%)	ASH (%)	CALCIUM (MG. PER 100 G.)	PHOSPHORUS (MG. PER 100 G).
Raw Meat	11.56–11.82	4.15–4.08	148–140	377–389
Cooked Meat	11.52–11.50	3.92–3.85	118–121	371–377
No Fertilizer	13.21–13.49	3.48–3.55	153–155	396–392

flabby and thin and feel much like tissue paper, but those fertilized with raw meat are firm and heavy in texture. Those on no fertilizer have leaves a little below the quality of the plants fertilized with raw meat.

One month after planting, all the beans are transplanted to larger plots. It is found that the roots of the plants fertilized with raw meat are at least twice as numerous, tougher, and longer than those of the others. The roots of the unfertilized plants are intermediate, but those of the plants fertilized with cooked meat are few, soft, and mushy.

The beans were analyzed for their moisture, ash, calcium, and phosphorus content. The results of the analysis are given in Table XIV.

Navy Bean Experiment—1940

The following year, a similar experiment is repeated. The seeds harvested from the plants fertilized with the excreta of cats fed raw meat are planted in a plot treated with composted manure from cats fed raw meat. The seeds harvested from plants fertilized with the excreta of cats fed cooked meat are planted in a plot treated with composted manure from cats fed cooked meat. Seeds from the unfertilized plants are planted again in an unfertilized plot. Two plots are added. One plot is planted with the seeds of the unfertilized beans in ground fertilized by the excreta of cats whose main diet consisted of pasteurized milk, and the other plot is planted with seeds of unfertilized beans in ground fertilized by the excreta of cats whose main diet was certified raw milk. This makes five plots in all: (1) raw meat, (2) cooked meat, (3) pasteurized milk, (4) certified raw milk, and (5) unfertilized.

In this experiment, the growth of the plants is similar to that of a year earlier. In the two plots fertilized with the excreta of cats on the milk diets, the beans of the certified raw milk group germinate sooner than the beans from the pasteurized milk group. The beans grown in the plot fertilized with the excreta of cats fed raw meat prove more even and regular in contour and in size. Their plants are sturdier, their color better, and the texture of their leaves superior to any of the other plants.

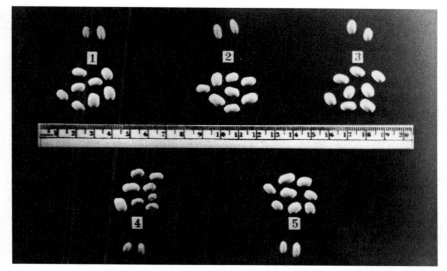

Fig. 13.5—Beans fertilized by composted cat manure and control: 1. Pasteurized milk; 2. Certified milk; 3. Raw meat; 4. Cooked meat; 5. No fertilizer.

Figure 13.5 shows the beans harvested from plants grown in plots fertilized by composted cat manure. The following is the breakdown of the findings:

Raw Meat: These beans have a hard white surface. Uniformity of size and plumpness of the beans distinguishes them from the beans of all other groups.

Cooked Meat: In this group, one-fourth of the beans are shriveled and are yellow in color; the remainder of the beans are smooth and white. They also are plumper than the milk beans, but they are not as plump as the beans fertilized with raw meat. They also exhibit the peculiar oblong shape of the beans fertilized with milk.

Pasteurized Milk: These beans have a hard, smooth white surface. The most noticeable features are their flatness and oblong shape.

Certified Raw Milk: These beans exhibit the same general features as those of the pasteurized group.

No Fertilizer: These beans are smooth and white. They are plumper than either of the beans fertilized with milk, but not as plump as the beans fertilized with meat.

There is a marked variation in the size and weight of the different groups of beans. Of the beans fertilized with pasteurized milk, the variation in

89

weight is from 72.2 mg to 198.3 mg with an average of 117.9 mg. In the group fertilized with certified raw milk, the variation is from 74.5 mg to 203 mg with an average of 121.7 mg. For the beans fertilized with raw meat, the smallest is 107 mg and the largest 210.4 mg with an average of 166.2 mg. For those fertilized with cooked meat, the smallest is 25.8 mg and the largest 209.9 mg with an average of 146.7 mg. The nonfertilized beans vary from 63.1 mg to 194.6 mg with an average of 113.5 mg.

A portion of the beans, the dried plants, and the pods, is subjected to chemical analysis. The results are given in Tables XV, XVI, and XVII.

TABLE XV. ANALYSIS OF NAVY BEANS: SECOND GENERATION

TYPE OF FERTILIZER USED ON NAVY BEANS	MOISTURE (%)	ASH (%)	CALCIUM (MG. PER 100 G.)	PHOSPHORUS (MG. PER 100 G).
Pasteurized Milk	12.78–12.97	4.33–4.30	80.2–78.8	489–478
Certified Milk	12.22–12.39	3.82–3.81	67.4–68.5	411–412
Raw Meat	12.91–12.97	414–412	131.0–130.0	448–449
Cooked Meat	12.54–12.61	3.94–3.92	87.5–89.0	455–457
No Fertilizer	12.51–12.66	4.15–4.03	83.1–86.3	490–487

TABLE XVI. ANALYSIS OF NAVY BEAN PLANTS: SECOND GENERATION

TYPE OF FERTILIZER USED ON NAVY BEANS	MOISTURE (%)	CRUDE FAT (%)	CRUDE FIBER (%)
Pasteurized Milk	8.90–8.92	5.11–5.21	35.84–35.44
Certified Milk	8.58–8.43	5.28–5.36	33.71–32.88
Raw Meat	8.68–8.56	5.82–5.54	35.81–35.74
Cooked Meat	7.70–7.71	9.21–9.73	27.01–26.92
No Fertilizer	8.88–8.71	5.81–5.80	27.50–27.67

TABLE XVII. ANALYSIS OF NAVY BEAN PODS: SECOND GENERATION

TYPE OF FERTILIZER USED ON NAVY BEANS	MOISTURE (%)	CRUDE FAT (%)	CRUDE FIBER (%)
Pasteurized Milk	9.61–9.73	14.15–14.43	26.89–27.33
Certified Milk	8.75–8.81	17.69–17.96	28.63–28.91
Raw Meat	11.29–11.57	15.29–15.39	28.54–28.27
Cooked Meat	7.19–7.16	24.82–25.22	29.89–30.31
No Fertilizer	11.04–10.81	13.64–13.37	26.70–27.05

No definite conclusions can be drawn from this experiment, but it suggests the possibility that excreta of diseased and healthy animals contain principles that affect plant growth, and that the health of the animal determines to some degree the effect on the vitality of the plant and its seeds as well as the chemical constituents of the plant, seed, and pod of the beans.

Chapter Fourteen

FAD DIETS AND OPTIMUM NUTRITION

"What We Know for Sure about an Optimal Diet for Human Beings"

The World Health Organization defines *health* as "a state of complete physical, mental and social well-being and not merely the absence of disease or infirmity." The National Research Council states that if optimum nutrition depends on optimum diet, "this becomes distinctly significant if one recognizes that health . . . has quantitative characteristics involving efficiency, reserves and the capacity not only to avoid diseases but to attain maximum inherited potentialities."

My own definition of an optimal diet is one that provides man with the nutrients essential to regenerate his body cells; to enable him to mature regularly as determined by normal osseous, physical, and mental characteristics; to resist disease; to reproduce his kind in homogeneity; and to enable him to produce a livelihood for himself and his family.

Healthy human beings have been known to fulfill these standards on various dietaries: (1) vegetarian with small amounts of eggs, milk, meat, or fish; (2) carnivorous, including fish, crustacea, mollusks, and small amounts of vegetation; and (3) omnivorous, including many combinations of vegetarian and carnivorous foods.

The American people have been great faddists about diet. What may be a medical necessity for some, frequently becomes a fad for others who are not in need of treatment. When I was a child, cod liver oil was considered essential for all children. The chemist discovered that other oils contained similar physical properties, and the cult of cod liver oil waned. About the time I entered medical school, salt was believed to cause high blood pressure, and some diets were restricted in salt; this belief waned only to revive recently. Meanwhile, chemists were able to concentrate vitamins A and D from fish livers, and vitamin preparations began their ascendancy and have remained popular as vitamin after vitamin has been synthesized. When dentists demonstrated that sugar caused tooth decay, there was a prompt decline in the use of sugar. One of the most recent fads is based on the assumption that excessive cholesterol is caused by foods, including animal fat, cream, butter, eggs, and by implication, all fats. Countering this is the discovery that unsaturated fatty acids, especially those found in vegetable oils and cold liver oil, reduce cholesterol in the blood stream.

Many women and young girls caught in the web of modern fashion for the slender silhouette have gone to great extremes in dieting. Without medical guidance, they have undertaken self-imposed diets providing as little as 700 to 900 calories a day. An alarming number of them are caught in the vicious circle of low energy, menstrual irregularity, poor skin, nervous exhaustion, irritability, frequent colds, anemia, and other unpredictable disorders. Such dieting is a perilous experience for women in their menopause. It is a far more perilous experience for developing girls and young women of child-bearing age. By upsetting their metabolism, they set the stage for difficult pregnancies and delicate infants.

Though it is medically possible to help the diet-starved woman, it is not simple. Their appetites may have failed, making a normal food intake a hardship. They may have diminished the enzyme content of their digestive juices, making food assimilation difficult. Consequently, they may require bed rest and a gradual program of feeding to build up their strength and their ability to exercise normally. I personally advocate a 3000 calorie diet with one part proteins, one part fat, of which 10 percent is unsaturated fatty acids, and one part carbohydrates.

In my experience, there is no more important time to insure that a diet is optimal than during pregnancy. The normal development of a fetus depends on the expectant mother's nutrition. Give her a diet of adequate nutrients, make sure that she is physically active without overtiring and that she is emotionally serene. She will soon feel the vigorous kicking of her baby *in utero* as her term nears its end.

I know for certain that breast milk from a healthy mother is the optimal diet for infants. If it is necessary to remove a baby from the breast before a normal span of nursing, or if nursing for some reason is not possible, I would place the infant on raw certified milk, where it is available. I would place the infant on raw liver and brain tissue after instructing the mother how to recognize healthy liver. I would not add muscle meat until the fifth or sixth month. Finally, I would let the baby chew on a chicken bone, when he can grasp it, to toughen his gums, and I would encourage his shoulder girdle development through programmed exercise. By the end of the first year, the child will be ready to eat some of the normal family fare and will be able to metabolize at least the recommended 1000 calories a day, and by the second year, 2000 calories a day.

The dietary goal we seek to fulfill is obviously different from that obtained by powdered or canned milk formulas with their canned fruit, vegetable, and meat supplements. We are working to develop hard muscles and tight ligaments. We are working for hearty appetites so that children can properly metabolize food and maintain an optimal development with strong resistance to disease.

We know for sure that if we are to be a nation of healthy human beings, self-confident in our abilities to meet life's challenges, we must start searching our souls for ways to insure that unborn generations of Americans can still obtain and metabolize an optimal diet.

Chapter Fifteen

THE IMPORTANCE OF FATS IN NUTRITION

"Essentiality of Fats in Nutrition," "In Defense of Fat," "The Therapeutic Value of a Thermolabile Factor Found in Fats, Particularly the Lecithins, In Dermatoses," "A Common Form of Fat Dyscrasia: Dry Skin"

Fats are present in each living cell and are essential to its life. The human body varies in fat content, but as an average figure, a 150-pound man is estimated to be composed of:

Body Weight	70 kg	100%
Fat	7 kg	10%
Protein	6.4 kg	9%
Carbohydrate	5.6 kg	8%
Mineral	2.0 kg	3%
Water	50.0 kg	70%

Intracellular fat is an important constituent in tissues such as muscle, brain, pancreas, and skin. Nerves are surrounded by a myelin sheath largely composed of fats; and the leukocytes, the life-protecting scavengers of our body, are also largely composed of fats.

The fat pads of the infant protect him from breaking his bones or impairing other parts of the body by acting as a cushion when he falls. Fat serves as a cushion and a support for the viscera. The pressure fat pads of the hands, especially over the metacarpal heads, are of the utmost importance to comfort while working. The pain caused by the loss of these pads can make work with tools difficult to impossible to perform. Similarly, the loss of the pads in the feet, especially those over the metatarsal heads and over the heels, may almost preclude walking.

Pressure pads are slow to replace once lost. Many never return. This is true of the ischial pads of the older person. Aging plays an important part in the loss of fat pads, either by design or altered metabolism. This makes the elderly more susceptible to mechanical injuries to joints, bones, and blood vessels. Furthermore, a person may be obese and yet have poor fat and, thus, poor pressure pads; however a muscular, skinny person may have excellent pressure fat pads regardless of age.

Subcutaneous fat aids an individual in resisting excessive environmental temperature changes. Fat forms a thermal barrier to prevent the body from losing heat when exposed to cold; and in case of excessive heat, a well-distributed subcutaneous adipose tissue may save a life or protect a vital organ.

The surface of the skin is protected by a very fine fatty secretion containing the unsaturated fatty acid fraction of the sebaceous secretion and other lipoid materials such as hormones and proteins. The ability of the unsaturated fatty acids to polymerize and to form flexible plastic surfaces provides the protective covering for the skin. The basic reaction involved is no different than that involved when the oxygen in the air polymerizes linseed oil to make a fine plastic surface for furniture.

Adequate fat intake not only provides the plastic surface covering for the skin, it provides the skin with bacteriacidal properties that prevent invasion by the myriad of surrounding pathological organisms. Likewise, the plastic layer prevents dirt and grime from penetrating the layers of the skin. Consequently, not only does insufficient intake of unsaturated fats produce a rough, unattractive skin, but it can cause the skin to develop painful cracks and abrasions.

Saturated and Unsaturated Fats

The primary source of man's fats is vegetable; the secondary source is animal. Fats, like proteins and carbohydrates, are of many types, but are primarily triglycerides, which are made up of fatty acids and phospholipids. The fatty acids may be either saturated or unsaturated, and the unsaturated fatty acids may be of one or more double bonds. The double-bonded fatty acids with 2 to 5 active radicals show the greater biological activity. The phospholipids, of which lecithin and cephalin are important members, are effective wetting agents, and one of their essential uses in the body is to mix water in oil and oil in water.

Essential fatty acids in foods can be harmful if allowed to become rancid. Their spontaneous change into odoriferous aldehydes, ketones, and esters spoils food. The problem of rancidity is one of preeminent concern to the food industry. However, in the processing and stabilizing of vegetable oils and cereal grains to avoid this problem, many of our finest sources of unsaturated fats have been rendered nutritively useless, except for the production of heat.

The prevailing fear of coronary disease causes people to avoid eating the fat of meats, though it is a valuable source of unsaturated fat. The butcher frequently cuts away a large share of the fat on a roast and on other cuts of meat. Those who do consume meat fats are apt to want them well cooked and crispy. When foods are cooked at high temperatures, many of the unsaturated fatty acids are oxidized at their double bonds, creating a different chemical of questionable metabolic value. It is known that when fats are heated to high temperature, the breakdown of glycerin produces acroline, a known poison. Lecithin, like other lipid substances, is subject to breakdown at normal cooking temperatures. Milk fats are also altered during heat processing, as in pasteurized cream and butter.

Fat is the energy fuel of the body. The potential rate of heat production is proportional to the degree of saturation of the fat. Though some of the fat we consume is immediately brought into new chemical relationships, much of it is stored in fatty deposits. The nature of this fat is dependent, in part, on the ingested fat. It is simple to change the character of bodily fat from soft to hard by increasing the intake of unsaturated fats.

In our experience, dry skin provides an index of disturbed fat metabolism. Most patients attribute their dry skin disorders to one of the following causes: hard water, improperly neutralized soaps, detergents, various household chemicals, exposure to the sun or wind, dry weather, dust, and incompatible or excessive cosmetics. Few suspect deficiencies in their fat intake. Recognizing that fatty acids have largely disappeared from our modern dietary, we have worked out a high protein, high fat, low carbohydrate diet for general rehabilitation. The diet prescribed includes liver and brain, cod liver oil, soybean lecithin, and edible linseed oil. In our experience, the conscientious patient usually shows skin improvements in one week and may recover completely within two months.

Chapter Sixteen

THE VALUE OF RAW FOOD AND GELATIN TO DIGESTION

"Hydrophilic Colloidal Diet"

Raw food consists largely of hydrophilic colloids, which are essential in the digestive process. Because of the hydration capacity of colloids, they absorb digestive juices and so prevent the common ailments of sour or acid stomach.

The heat used in cooking foods precipitates their colloids, alters their hydration capacity, and interferes with the digestive process. The amount of interference depends upon the degree of heat used and upon the specific character of the colloidal medium itself. Certain colloids will withstand more heat than others; for instance, cellulose of vegetable origin and certain pectins will stand a greater temperature without precipitating colloids than proteins of animal origin.

Any hydrophilic colloid, be it living protoplasm or a mineral jell, has a specific hydration capacity under given conditions. By varying the physiochemical condition surrounding a colloid, it can be made to expand or contract. For instance, if two gelatin squares of similar weight are immersed in bowls, one containing distilled water, the other a solution of hydrochloric acid of 1/100 normal concentration, two things happen. First, the gelatin square in the acid expands at a much greater rate than the square in water. Second, the solution surrounding the square in the acid medium becomes almost the same hydrogen ion concentration as distilled water. Now, if the acid solution is made stronger, the gelatin is digested making a colloidal suspension, and unless too great a concentration of acid is present, the acidity of the solution approaches neutrality. On the other hand, gelatin precipitated by heat fails to take up water or acid.

If man did not cook his food, there would be no need for the addition of any hydrophilic colloid to his dietary. Uncooked foods contain sufficient hydrophilic colloids to keep gastric mucosa in excellent condition. As we live largely on cooked food, problems arise. An old description of the stomach contents portrays them in layers, each layer assuming its position by virtue of its specific gravity: meat first, then vegetables and fruits, followed by and interspersed with mashed potatoes, and finally the water layer with its scum of fat. According to this view, these layers churn around in sufficient gastric juices to digest the meal in one and one-half hours to four hours, if all goes well. If these gastric contents are then removed and examined, the aqueous layer is strongly acid, though the degree of acidity differs with the individual.

If we add a hydrophilic colloid of excellent hydration capacity to the diet portrayed above, a definite change takes place in the stomach contents. If they are withdrawn for analysis, a gluey mass is recovered. It is not sour as are the stomach contents without the gelatin; it does not show any acidity until the colloid is broken down. Under these conditions, digestion is generally distributed throughout the mass rather than layered.

When raw fruits and vegetables are eaten, they first absorb the digestive juices and are partially digested before the gluey mass develops. Raw meats apparently become gelatinous in less time than vegetables, but as digestion proceeds, all raw food becomes more or less gelatinous before liquification takes place. When cooked foods are eaten, gastric digestion may be interfered with because the heat of cooking precipitates colloids. Gelatin, because of its availability and relatively low cost, can act as a supplemental hydrophilic colloid for dietary usage in combating disturbances caused by cooked food.

Chapter Seventeen

THE HIGH PROTECTIVE DIET

"The Importance of a Vital, High Protective Diet in the Treatment of Tuberculosis and Allied Conditions," "The Patient Manual"

The food habits of our population have undergone a marked change in the last decades. The amount of carbohydrate consumed has been increasing steadily with subsequent decrease in the consumption of fats and protein, particularly the latter. People have become vitamin conscious, and in trying to obtain the necessary amounts of these compounds, have neglected other food elements that are essential.

How many people are aware that a high caloric intake is essential for maintaining body equilibrium? This is a fact that is not emphasized, but the fact that sugar and starches give quick energy is receiving undue emphasis. From the standpoint of energy, proteins have the highest specific dynamic action. Gram for gram, fats furnish two and one-quarter times as much energy as carbohydrates.

The High Protective Diet we give our patients is one part protein, one part fat, and one part carbohydrate. There are four principles to this diet:

1. Food is altered as little as possible by using minimal temperatures in cooking.
2. Vitamins are obtained from foods naturally rich in them.
3. Minerals are supplied by the use of relatively crude foodstuffs and by a mineral salt preparation.
4. Gelatin, a hydrophilic colloid, is used as a regular part of the diet because it aids digestion.

For the average adult, the diet is planned to provide 225 grams each of protein, fat, and carbohydrates. The carbohydrates recommended here are in whole grains, unrefined sweets, the starches of vegetables, and in meats. For children, cut down the portions and give second helpings rather than overwhelming them with one large serving.

Basic Instructions

1. Cook in stainless steel, enamelware, ironware, or glass. Do not use pressure cookers.
2. Use drinking water liberally. Estimate the total intake of fluids per day at one pint to 20 pounds of body weight for adults.
3. Use the mineral salt mixture for table salt.
4. Use a variety of spices for food interest, for stimulating the appetite, and for producing gastric juices.
5. Use gelatin three times a day. (See Recipe A)
6. Use animal fats, lard, and meat drippings instead of vegetable fats.
7. Use butter, not substitutes.
8. Pickle your foods. The use of vinegar and pickles in hot weather helps counteract ill effects of heat and also aids in maintaining good gastric acidity.
9. When children are old enough to have a general diet, allow them to have pickles.
10. Use soups daily. (See Recipe F)

Breakfast pattern:

Sliced orange or half of a grapefruit
4 prunes or figs
1 glass of whole raw milk
1 glass gelatin drink
1 cup coffee or tea (adults)
Bacon or ham with an egg or lamb chop
1 bowl of whole grain hot cereal with cream and without sugar

Luncheon pattern:

Hot soup (if hot vegetable soup, serve the soup meat as well)
One of the variety meats (if soup meat is not served) (8 oz.)
Generous portion of mixed green salad
One hot vegetable
1 glass of milk
1 glass of gelatin drink
1 serving of whole grain bread with butter
Dessert

Dinner pattern:

> Raw beef hors d'oeuvres (three times weekly)
> Plain hot soup, such as chicken broth or bouillon
> Roast of other cut of meat (8 oz.)
> Green salad (mixed green, if this has not been served at noon)
> 2 hot vegetables, one of which is yellow
> 1 glass milk
> 1 glass gelatin drink
> Dessert

Note: The luncheon and dinner patterns are somewhat interchangeable. Where meat substitutes, such as dried beans and cheese, are planned, make sure to add additional proteins, such as leftover meats, eggs, or fish.

Milk and Dairy Products

1. Use clean, unprocessed milk. Know your dairy and the health record of the herd. If you do not, buy certified milk, which must meet the highest state and county safety requirements.
2. Use unprocessed cheeses. Use no renovated cheeses.

Eggs

1. Use fertile eggs of hatching quality for eating because they contain natural estrogenic substances.
2. Vary the methods of preparation of breakfast eggs to maintain interest.

Cereals and Breadstuffs

1. Use only whole grain cereals.
2. Use whole grain flour instead of white.
3. Use 1 teaspoon of unprocessed 100% wheat germ with the breakfast cereal. Heat-treated wheat germ is of little value.
4. Use whole grain breadstuffs. The best are those you make in your own kitchen from freshly ground flours.

Beverages

1. For adults, restrict coffee and tea to one cup without sugar at breakfast time. In problems of asthma, use Postum or other substitute,

reserving coffee for its medicinal value. If gastric problems are present, eliminate entirely.
2. For both children and adults, use one glass of milk each meal.
3. Avoid soft drinks, which are nutritionally valueless, provide excess calories, and endanger the teeth.

Meats

1. Buy only government-inspected meats.
2. Use glandular or variety meats as one-third the necessary protein.
3. Grind your own beef. Grind only enough for immediate use since rapid oxidation may cause stomach distress.
4. Use the following meats rare: steaks, lamb chops, leg of lamb, rib and sirloin tip roasts, fresh ground beef for patties.
5. Fry meats only occasionally. Take care not to heat the fat to smoking since this causes the formation of chemical compounds that interfere with digestion.
6. Serve liver prepared according to Recipe B at last three times a week.
7 Serve brain eggnog (Recipe C) once or twice a week.
8. Serve pork rarely, except bacon.
9. Serve freshly ground beef (Recipe D) three times a week.
10. Use moderate heat for roasting meat, and salt when nearly done.
11. Simmer tough cuts of meat over low heat.
12. Serve fish roe, fish, and poultry often.

Vegetables

1. Purchase vegetables the days they are freshly brought to the market.
2. Wash quickly in running water, dry, store in refrigerator.
3. Use starchy vegetables such as potatoes and sweet potatoes no more than once a week; bake or steam in the jackets to preserve the minerals.
4. Use dry beans no more than twice a month. To enhance their portion value, sprout before cooking. (Recipe G)
5. Consume green leafy vegetables once each day as a salad.
6. Use a yellow vegetable once a day.
7. Cook green vegetables by steaming only until tender, by cooking in a small amount of water until tender, by sautéing quickly in butter or drippings. Reserve leftover juices for the soup kettle. Salt the vegetables after they have cooked, using mineral salt.

8. Use frozen vegetables in preference to canned.
9. Sprout mung beans, alfalfa seeds, and other seeds to obtain the highest vegetable protein. Use them in mixed green salads. (Recipe G)

Fruits

1. Use fresh fruits in season.
2. Thoroughly wash the skins of apples, pears, and other fruits to remove as well as possible any sprays. Wash all fruits quickly and store in refrigerator.
3. Serve citrus fruits whole instead of as a juice. When they are not available, serve tomato juice.
4. Serve frozen rather than canned fruits.
5. Serve raw pineapple occasionally.

Desserts

1. Use simple puddings, custard, jello, tapioca, home-made ice cream, cornstarch pudding, rice custard.
2. Cut down the sugar content to the bare minimum to give flavor.
3. Wherever the molasses flavor is desirable, as in whole grain steamed puddings, use unsulphured molasses in place of refined sugar. Use unpasteurized honey in small amounts for sweetening.
4. Serve fresh fruits in season, taking care that the protein need is first satisfied. Do not overeat fruits as they are heavy in sugar.
5. Make only those pastries that can be made of whole grain flours and minimal sweetening.
6. Eliminate candies.

Recipe A—Gelatin

Soak one tablespoon of plain gelatin in a cup with sufficient water to cover. Dissolve in a hot liquid such as soup, or hot water with fruit flavoring, or hot water in which a beef cube has been dissolved. Serve this faithfully with each meal.

Recipe B—Liver

Wash liver in cold water; dry on soft paper. Remove skin and tough fibers with a very sharp knife. Freeze. If the liver is light colored or spongy, discard, since it is unfit for eating.

Grate two tablespoons of the frozen liver; stir it quickly into a glass of cold tomato juice; season with catsup, horseradish, or other seasoning; salt and pepper; and consume at once.

This raw liver cocktail may be consumed in mid-morning, mid-afternoon, or as part of the meal.

A good variation of the raw liver is a cocktail, served as one would serve a fish cocktail: dice 2 ounces of liver into very small cubes, mix with slivers of green onion and diced celery, dress with well-seasoned mayonnaise in which a spoonful of cocktail sauce has been stirred, garnish with a slice of lemon.

Recipe C—Brains

Wash brains in cold water, remove membranes, rinse, and freeze. Grate 3 tablespoons of the brains on a very fine grater; beat the yolk of one egg with 3 ounces of 50-50 cream, add brains, season with a pinch of salt, add ¼ teaspoon of vanilla, and fold in the stiffly beaten egg white. Sprinkle nutmeg on the top. Serve before bedtime as a nightcap.

Use raw brains in salad:

1 c. hot water	½ c. cold water
1 tbsp. gelatin	¼ c. lime or lemon juice
1 tbsp. honey	1 set of cleaned brains

Place hot water in blender. Put lid on blender, turn on, and carefully add gelatin while running. Add honey, lime juice, and cold water. Pour gelatin mixture into mold. Cut brains in half-inch pieces with scissors. Add to gelatin mixture after it cools. Chill until set, slice, and serve on lettuce with mayonnaise.

Scrambled brains:

1 set of brains	2 tbsp. chopped parsley
1 tbsp. butter	salt
4 eggs	2 tbsp. milk

Parboil brains gently. Drain. Sauté gently in butter until browned. Add eggs to milk and beat, lightly scramble, and garnish with parsley.

Recipe D—Fresh Ground Beef

Grind 2 tablespoons of fresh beef with a little of its fat, spread on Ryekrisp or other breadstuff, salt and pepper, and use as an hors d'oeuvre at least three times a week.

Recipe E—Variety Meats Other than Liver and Brains

Sweetbreads: Soak fresh sweetbreads in cold water with one tablespoon of vinegar for half an hour. Parboil gently for 20 minutes; remove membranes when cool.

When thus prepared, sauté lightly in butter, or make a medium white sauce with cornstarch, cover with buttered crumbs, bake until heated through in the oven.

Kidneys: Trim, cut kidneys in half, remove white tubes, and soak in salted water for an hour.

When so prepared, use any favorite kidney recipe of your own or one of the following:

Kidney Sauté:

 1 beef kidney
 1 slice of ham
 2 medium onions

Brown ham. Cut kidney into one-inch squares. Drop into briskly boiling water for one minute; drain and rinse. Roll in whole wheat flour, salt, and pepper. Quickly fry with sliced onions and serve with the ham, piping hot.

Steak and Kidney Pie: Clean kidneys as directed above; cut into cubes, place in kettle of cold water, bring to a boil, discard water, and repeat a second time. Meanwhile, cut 1 pound of steak into 1¼ inch cubes, dredge with whole wheat flour, season with salt and pepper, and brown in heavy iron kettle in ¼ c. butter or drippings. Add chopped onion, 1 tsp. Worcestershire Sauce, cover with cold water, add kidneys, and simmer gently about 2 hours. Add liquid as needed, and stir to prevent sticking. Pour into casserole, top with a flaky crust made of whole wheat pastry flour, bake quickly, and serve very hot.

Heart: Cut out tough fibers, wash thoroughly in cold water.

Sautéed Heart: Slice calf's heart into one-inch slices crosswise. Roll in whole wheat flour, season with salt and pepper. Brown as you would chicken. Cover with cold water and simmer gently until tender. Add onion for flavor.

Baked Stuffed Heart: After cleaning beef heart, simmer for 2 hours in salted water. Prepare a bread stuffing, stuff the boiled heart, and skewer together. Roll in whole wheat flour, brown in bacon fat, place in covered casserole. Add a small amount of water to pan in which heart was browned, pour it over the heart, and bake slowly in moderate oven until tender.

Tripe: Select pickled or fresh tripe that has already been cooked, or simmer uncooked tripe, thoroughly washed, for 6 hours or until tender. Let cool in broth.

Fried Tripe: Cut cooked tripe into serving pieces. Dip in egg and crumbs and allow to dry before frying. Brown nicely in bacon fat and serve very hot.

Savory Tripe: Cut prepared tripe into inch squares, add onions, carrots, celery, bay leaf, peppercorns, a tablespoon of Worcestershire Sauce, and simmer about 25 minutes.

Recipe F—Soup

1. Once each week, make a large kettle of soup stock. Use plenty of bones, such as shank and knuckle, which should be split and the marrow browned, with whatever meat is used—shank, short-ribs, ox-tail, lamb trimmings or any inexpensive cut of meat. Cover the bones and meat with cold water, let stand for an hour before beginning to simmer. To extract the calcium from the bone, add ¼ cup of vinegar, and sufficient salt to flavor. *Simmer* until the meat falls from the bone. The browning of the meat and marrow will supply a brown color as well as a good flavor. Strain through a cloth. Cool, skim off the grease, which can be reserved for seasoning. Clear by pouring into the strained broth two slightly beaten egg whites, the shells, and two tablespoons of cold water; bring soup to a full boil for five minutes, then restrain. When cool, store the broth in the refrigerator. As an introduction to the noon or evening meal, heat sufficient broth for the one meal, adding vegetable juices or small amounts of cooked vegetables for variation. Always season the soup well and serve very hot.
2. Use any of the above meats with some bone to make a kettle of vegetable soup. When the meat is almost tender, add vegetables cut rather small, such as celery, onions, turnips, carrots, or any combination, with a bouquet of herbs, cooking the vegetables only until tender.
3. Cream soups of any vegetable, using cornstarch or whole wheat pastry flour to make the thickening, make excellent cool-weather soups.

Recipe G—Sprouting Beans and Grains

Mung bean sprouts: Wash ½ c. of seeds, soak overnight. Spread in the middle of a clean old bath towel, fold over the sides, roll up loosely, and soak with cold water. Lay on a wire rack over a bowl so that air circulates freely on all sides. Keep damp by sprinkling. Sprouts of good growth will be obtained in 3–5 days. Wash the sprouts to remove as many hulls as possible, and use the sprouts as part of a tossed salad. Or combine with meats to make chop-suey.

Use similar treatment on navy or kidney beans. When they are sprouted, cook them with ham or bacon fat. They will cook in a much shorter time than unsprouted beans, and will be practically free of the gas factor.

Alfalfa and clover seeds make excellent sprouts for salad.

There are porous crocks now on the market with lids, which are designed for sprouting seeds easily. They eliminate the use of the towel.

Appendix I

Biography of
Francis Marion Pottenger, Jr.

Francis Marion Pottenger, Sr., a native of Ohio, moved to Monrovia, California, in 1895 with his wife, who was suffering from tuberculosis. He entered into the practice of medicine, but when his wife's health failed to improve, he took her back to Ohio where she died in November of 1898. Returning to Monrovia, in 1903 he and his two brothers, Milton and Joseph, opened the Pottenger Sanatorium and Clinic for Diseases of the Chest, with an emphasis on the treatment of tuberculosis. Convinced that good nutrition formed the basis for the successful treatment of disease, Francis senior placed a priority on the quality of food he served at the sanatorium. Most of the food was grown on the premises, and to insure the best quality milk and milk products, he worked with the United States Department of Agriculture to form the first government-accredited (free of tuberculosis) Holstein herd in California. The sanatorium soon became recognized internationally for its successful treatment of tuberculosis and maintained an impeccable reputation until it closed in 1956. Francis wrote well over 200 books and articles on the treatment of chest diseases, many of which were used in medical schools throughout the country.

Francis senior married his second wife, Adelaide Gertrude Babbit (Kitty), on August 29, 1900. Kitty was a native of Keysville, New York, and at the time of their courtship was the vice principal and teacher of Latin and Greek in the Monrovia High School. The Babbit family was known for its inventors. One Babbit ancestor invented Babbit metal, an alloy used in the production of bearings. The metal was developed for the New Haven Railroad in order to circumvent the British monopoly on replacement parts for their locomotives. Another Babbit invention was Babbo, a popular household cleaning agent and the predecessor of today's Ajax.

Three children were born of the union between Francis and Kitty: Francis Marion, Jr., on May 29, 1901; Robert Thomas in 1904; and Adelaide Marie in 1907. The family home, called the Oaks, was built by W. N. Monroe, the founder of Monrovia. The Oaks was also a working farm and provided both farming experience for the children and fresh food for the family table.

Francis Marion Pottenger, Jr., began his schooling at the Wild Rose Elementary School in Monrovia. Here he made many permanent friends. One was Thomas Myron Hotchkiss, who wrote a biography of Francis in which he describes Francis's early inventive talent. "When we were boys, 'Meccano' sets were all the rage, and Francis had a rather elaborate set. With it he made a working model of a rock crusher such as were found in the Azusa-Duarte area where the gravel resources of the San Gabriel River were being exploited by rock companies. He set his model up in the foyer of the Old Wild Rose School where it was enviously eyed by many of his companions. Later, with the same set he constructed a working model of a bascule bridge complete with motor drive. Both models displayed considerable ingenuity in design and construction."

In his teens, Francis pursued his interest in mechanical and electrical invention by developing a system of tractor-drawn, heated meal carts to deliver hot meals from the sanatorium kitchen to the outlying patient cottages. According to Francis's diary, he met many frustrations and spent much time repairing the tractors and carts, as well as overcoming other maintenance problems. His persistence paid off, however, and his meal delivery system worked and was used until the closing of the sanatorium.

When Francis finished Wild Rose School, he attended Monrovia High School, Los Angeles Military Academy, the Claremont School for Boys (Webb School), and Thatcher in Ojai Valley. This shifting of schools was due in part to intermittent poor health. During his growing years, he suffered chronic otitis media and mastoiditis and was forced to spend two to three months out of every school year in bed. Prior to entering college, he spent nearly three years in bed, making Cottage 80 at the sanatorium his home away from home.

Francis's formal education during this time was largely supervised by members of his family as well as by tutors. Though he took many correspondence courses, he became accustomed to a personalized, Socratic method of learning and maintained a lifelong preference for gaining knowledge by conversing with the experts in his various fields of interest rather than by reading.

Though his natural inclination was towards engineering, his father insisted that be become a physician. Accordingly, Francis entered his father's alma mater, Otterbein College in Westerville, Ohio, in 1921. Here he met Teresa Elizabeth Saxour and on the day of their graduation, June 17, 1925, they were married. Francis proceeded to College of Medicine at the University of Cincinnati, also his father's medical school. He received his M.B. in 1929, which allowed him to practice medicine in Ohio. In 1920, he received his M.D. and began his internship at the Los Angeles County Hospital.

During these preparatory years at Otterbein and at medical school, Francis kept extensive notes of his observations and the questions raised by them. His notebook reveals the wide range of his early introspective searchings:

"Is it not probable that the fineness of the hair may be indication of the thickness of the skin?" 3/14/25

"Why is malignancy rare in the duodenum?" 1/19/28

"Is hunger caused by the deprivation of body tissues of carbohydrates?" 1/27/28

"Is it possible that cancer may be produced by intestinal bacteria which liberate an enzyme that has power to cause the cells of specific tissues to proliferate—the tissues being in such a state that trauma starts the proliferation?"

His earliest contributions to medical literature appeared in the *Journal of the American Medical Association* in November of 1930 when he was still interning at the Los Angeles County Hospital. In two articles, he describes his inventions of "Rubber Flask Connectors for Hypodermoclysis, Intravenous Therapy and Other Uses" and "A New Siphon System for Maintaining Continuous Drainage Without Air Block in Thoracic Emphyemas and in Infections of Other Body Cavities." The latter system, known as Pottenger suction, was adopted by the Chest Surgery Section of the Los Angeles County Hospital and was used for many years until mechanical pumps came into wide use.

While he was attending medical school, he developed a "hatred" for the way civilized man treated himself and his children. He wondered why people, so capable of advancing their technology, failed so miserably in promoting their biological health. He felt a driving need to know and to understand how man could maintain good health and eliminate chronic illness and so prevent children from suffering as he had. This missionary zeal led him to direct his inquiry toward the field of nutrition.

On completing his internship, he became a resident physician at the sanatorium and, in 1931, became a vice president of the corporation and associate medical director and the director of research for the Pottenger Sanatorium and Clinic. During the 1930s, Francis began his own research into the treatment of tuberculosis and other respiratory ailments, such as asthma. He became interested in Drs. Pfiffner and Swingle's work with adrenal glands and began conducting experiments feeding adrenal hormones to tuberculous guinea pigs. In 1937, he published a paper with his Uncle, Joseph Pottenger, in which he showed that, in 28 percent of the guinea pigs treated with adrenal extracts, there was no evidence of tuberculosis when they were sacrificed for pathological study.

At this time, he also started a small private practice using the sanatorium's facilities, but soon considered the possibility of founding his own clinic. He did not have to look far for a suitable site. At the end of the First World War, the Pottenger Sanatorium had been compelled to expand in order to care for returning veterans with pulmonary problems from gas poisoning and infections. Several cottages were built off the main grounds, and as the case load of veterans began to drop, these cottages fell into disuse. Francis purchased them, and after extensive remodeling, he opened the Francis M. Pottenger, Jr., Hospital for the treatment of nontuberculous diseases of the respiratory system, with a particular emphasis on asthma. The opening was in 1940, and the 42-bed hospital operated until 1960.

Continuing his research into the therapeutic use of adrenal hormones, Francis began treating his asthmatic patients with a high protein diet supplemented by freshly ground adrenal glands. This treatment brought marked improvement to most of his patients and led him to make a major commitment to the manufacture of his own adrenal extract, known to his patients as "X06." He designed and built an extracting and refrigerating facility with a walk-in, room-sized freezer, one of the first of its kind. His patent for this facility had nine separate claims.

In the 1930s and 1940s, biological extracts were assayed and standardized by their effects on other biological systems, usually laboratory animals. Francis used cats to determine the hormone content of his adrenal extract. Removing their adrenal glands, he gave them supportive doses of his newly manufactured extracts in order to observe their reactions. Through his observations, he was able to determine the strength of each batch of extract and to obtain the necessary uniformity in potency. It was this process of biological standardization that led to his ten-year cat study.

Prior to his death in 1967, Francis was involved in developing photographic and X-ray equipment capable of giving simultaneous exposures and an accurate superimposition of the X-ray and photograph. He planned to investigate the changes in human anatomy over a span of four generations, roughly from 1900, 1920, 1940, and to 1960. The study was to consist of X-rays of the skull, hand, foot, and thorax of 7000 individuals, with corresponding anthropometric photographs and measurements. His preliminary findings were revealing that dramatic changes had occurred in the anatomy of the American male from a turn-of-the-century figure with broad shoulders, stocky neck, and narrow hips to a modern figure with small, weak shoulders, longer neck, and broad pelvis. The reverse development was appearing in the anatomy of the American female with a 1900 figure showing narrow shoulders and broad pelvis to a 1960 figure showing broad shoulders and a narrow pelvis.

Francis was among the first in his profession to recognize the health hazard of air pollution in Los Angeles County. He worked tirelessly to alert responsible parties to the toxic properties of smog. As a consequence of his efforts, he was appointed to the Los Angeles Air Pollution Control District's Scientific Committee on Air Pollution and was a member of the Air Pollution Committee of the College of Chest Physicians.

He also was among the first to recognize the hazards of pesticides to human health. In a paper entitled "Poisoning from DDT and Other Chlorinated Hydrocarbon Pesticides," he stated: "The widespread use of chlorinated hydrocarbons such as DDT in agriculture, animal husbandry and about the home has been accompanied by a syndrome of hepatic and neurologic damage and sometimes death." This paper presented the first reported cases of insecticide poisoning. He defined the symptoms as (1) hyperirritability, anxiety, confusion, inability to concentrate, forgetfulness, as well as slow or racing heartbeats; (2) pathological liver hypertrophy, renal lesions, loss of colloid in the thyroid, and changes in nerve and skin tissues; and (3) the presence of insecticide in the body's fat deposits.

In the 1940s, Francis became acquainted with Dr. Weston A. Price, a practicing dentist with a congenial spirit of inquiry. In his desire to explain the prevalence of tooth decay and facial inadequacies among his patients and "civilized peoples," Price set upon a worldwide odyssey to study the dietary habits of fourteen isolated and primitive peoples. He found that those natives who still ate their customary natural foods—whether primarily fish, meat, or vegetable—showed broad facial structures, a "perfection" to their dental arches, and virtually no tooth decay; however, those who had been exposed to the civilized diet of commerce based on refined white sugar, white flour, canned and packaged foods, showed narrowing of their faces, crowding of their teeth, and a high incidence of cavities. They also showed increasing susceptibility to tuberculosis and other degenerative diseases.

Appreciating the importance of Weston Price's findings and their confirmation of his own experimental and clinical findings, Francis became chairman of a committee established for the purpose of disseminating Price's work through exhibits, lectures, and printed materials. Later, The Weston A. Price Memorial Foundation was organized as a nonprofit organization to further this educational purpose. At his death, Francis's extensive library of research data, slides, X-ray studies, papers, and articles were entrusted to the foundation by his family. In response, the Board of Directors changed the foundation's name to The Price-Pottenger Nutrition Foundation, disseminating the work of both men. The name was simplified to Price-Pottenger in 2016, reflecting the wide appeal the foundation has achieved.

During his professional career, Francis wrote many articles, which appeared in different medical publications. Appendix II lists these papers and articles. One of his favorite, unpublished stories took place at a nutrition meeting he was attending.

A reporter came up to him and asked, "Are all these people here interested in nutrition?"

Francis answered, "Yes."

The reporter commented, "They certainly are not a very healthy looking crowd."

To which Francis replied quizzically, "Why do you think we are here?"

Francis and Elizabeth had four children: Francis Marion, III, Margaret Elizabeth, Barbara Jane, and Samuel Slatter. Francis III received his doctorate in education and is presently supervising the curriculum for the public school system in Hawaii. Margaret is the owner of two dress stores called The Jabberwocky in Tustin, California. Barbara lives with her lawyer husband, Jim Shumar, in Whitacre, Virginia. Samuel is deceased.

Francis's younger brother, Robert Thomas, practiced medicine in Pasadena, California. In addition to promoting the importance of optimal nutrition, Robert pioneered clinical research in the area of food allergy in the treatment and control of arthritis and rheumatism. The authors of this monograph are the son and daughter of Robert. Robert Thomas Pottenger, Jr., is a practicing physician in Pasadena and continues the tradition of his father and uncle in his own research and clinical practice. Elaine Pottenger is a writer.

Appendix II

THE PROFESSIONAL PAPERS OF
FRANCIS M. POTTENGER, JR., M.D.

1. Rubber Flask Connectors for Hypodermoclysis, Intravenous Therapy and Other Uses. *Journal of the American Medical Association*, November 1930.
2. A New Siphon System for Maintaining Continuous Drainage Without Air Block in Thoracic Empyemas and in Infections of Other Body Cavities. *Journal of the American Medical Association*, November 1930.
3. The Treatment of Asthma. *California and Western Medicine*, July 1935, Vol. 43, No. 1. (With F. M. Pottenger, M.D., and Robert T. Pottenger, M.D.)
4. Clinical and Experimental Evidence of Growth Factors in Raw Milk. *Certified Milk*, January 1937.
5. Evidence of the Protective Influences of Adrenal Hormones Against Tuberculosis in Guinea Pigs. *Endocrinology*, July 1937, Vol. 21, No. 4, pp. 529–532. (With J. E. Pottenger, M.D.)
6. A Male Sex-Stimulating and Female Sex-Repressive Fraction from the Adrenal Gland. *Endocrinology*, February 1938, Vol. 22, No. 2, pp. 197–202. (With D. G. Simonsen, Ph.D.)
7. Hydrophilic Colloidal Diet. *American Journal of Digestive Diseases*, April 1938, Vol 5, No. 2, pp. 96–99.
8. Clinical Evidences of the Value of Raw Milk. *Certified Milk*, July 1938.
9. An Orally-Active Sex-Maturation Fraction from the Adrenal Gland. *Endocrinology*, February 1938, Vol. 22, No. 2, pp. 203–206. (With D. G. Simonsen, Ph.D.)
10. The Use of the Adrenal Cortex in the Treatment of the Common Cold. *Medical Record*, February 16, 1938.
11. Adrenal Cortex in Treating Childhood Asthma: Clinical Evaluation of its Use. *California and Western Medicine*, October 1938, Vol. 49, No. 4. (With F. M. Pottenger, M.D.)
12. Deficient Calcification Produced by Diet: Experimental and Clinical Considerations. *Transactions of American Therapeutic Society*, 1939. (With D. G. Simonsen, Ph.D.)
13. Further Studies of Male Sex-Stimulating, Female Sex-Repressive Fractions of the Adrenal Gland of Cows, Steers and Bulls. *Endocrinology*, February 1939, Vol. 24, No. 2, pp. 187–193. (With D. G. Simonsen, Ph.D.)
14. The Influence of Heat Labile Factors on Nutrition in Oral Development and Health. *Journal of Southern California State Dental Association*, November 1939. (With D. G. Simonsen, Ph.D.)
15. Heat Labile Factors Necessary for the Proper Growth and Development of Cats. *Journal of Laboratory and Clinical Medicine*, December 1939, Vol. 25, No. 6, pp. 238–240.

16. The Clinical Significance of the Osseous System. *Transactions of the American Therapeutic Society*, 1940, Vol. 40.

17. The Demonstration of Mycobacterium Tuberculosis in Anorectal Abscess. *Surgery, Gynecology and Obstetrics*, May 1941, Vol. 72, pp. 936–938. (With J. E. Pottenger, M.D.)

18. The Importance of a Vital, High Protein Diet in the Treatment of Tuberculosis and Allied Conditions. *Bulletin of the American Academy of Tuberculosis Physicians*, July 1941.

19. The Reciprocal Relationship of the Health of Plants, Animals and Human Beings.

20. Nutritional Aspects of the Orthodontic Problem. *The Angel Orthodontist*, October 1942, Vol. 12, No. 4.

21. Disappearance of Tuberculin Reaction in Children Under Treatment for Allergies.

22. The Therapeutic Value of a Thermolabile Factor Found in Fats, Particularly the Lecithins, in Dermatoses. *Transactions of the American Therapeutic Society*, 1943. *Southern Medical Journal*, April 1944, Vol. 37, pp. 211–216.

23. Studies of Fragmentation of the Tarsal and Metatarsal Bones Resulting from Recurrent Metabolic Insults. *Transactions of the American Therapeutic Society*, 1945, Vol. 45.

24. Fragmentation and Scarring of the Tarsal and Metatarsal Bones: An Index of Dental Deformity. *Journal of Orthodontics and Oral Surgery*, August 1946, Vol. 32, No. 8, pp. 486–515.

25. The Effect of Heat-Processed Foods and Metabolized Vitamin D Milk on the Dentofacial Structures of Experimental Animals. *Journal of Orthodontics and Oral Surgery*, August 1946, Vol. 32, No. 8, pp. 467–485.

26. Adequate Diet in Tuberculosis. *American Review of Tuberculosis*, September 1946, Vol. 54, No. 3. (With F. M. Pottenger, M.D.)

27. The Responsibility of the Pediatrician in the Orthodontic Problem. *California Medicine*, October 1946, Vol. 65, No. 4.

28. Brucella Infections. *Merck Report*, July 1949. (With Ira Allison and Wm. A. Albrecht, Ph.D.)

29. The Use of Copper, Cobalt, Manganese and Iodine in the Treatment of Undulant Fever. *Annals of Western Medicine and Surgery*, September 1949.

30. A Common Form of Fat Dyscrasia: Dry Skin. *Southern Medical Journal*, February 1950, Vol. 43, No. 2.

31. The Use of a Readily Available Vegetable Material in the Treatment of Arthrides. *Transactions of the American Therapeutic Society*, April 1950.

32. Influence of Breast Feeding on Facial Development. *Archives of Pediatrics*, October 1950, Vol. 67, pp. 454–461. (With Bernard Krohn, M.D.)

33. Emergency Treatment of the Asthmatic with Special Reference to Adrenal Cortex & Vit. B12. *Rocky Mountain Medical Journal*, April 1951. (With Bernard Krohn, M.D.)

34. The Effects of Disturbed Nutrition on Dentofacial Structures. *Southern California State Dental Journal*, February 1952.

35. Allergic Rhinitis Tocopherol Therapy. *Annals of Western Medicine and Surgery*, August 1952, Vol. 6, No. 8, pp. 484–487. (With Bernard Krohn, M.D.)

36. Providing an Adequate Diet. *Journal of the Tennessee State Dental Association*, Jan. 1952, Vol. 32, No. 1, pp. 29–32.

37. Reduction of Hypercholesterolemia by High Fat Diet Plus Soybean Phospholipids. *American Journal of Digestive Diseases*, April 1953, Vol. 19, No. 4, pp. 107–109. (With Bernard Krohn, M.D.)

38. Essentiality of Fats in Nutrition. *Journal of Applied Nutrition*, Autumn 1956, Vol. 9, No. 2, pp. 394–397.

39. Therapeutic Effect of Lamb Fat in the Dietary. *Journal of Applied Nutrition*, Spring 1957, Vol. 10, No. 2.

40. Dietary Rehabilitation of the Malnourished. *General Practice*, June 1957, Vol. 20, No. 6.

41. In Defense of Fat. *General Practice*, July 1957, Vol. 20, No 7.

43. The Effect of Diet on the Nutrition of the Dental Patient. *Southern California State Dental Assistants Journal*, February 1959.

43. What We Know for Sure about an Optimal Diet for Human Beings. *Clinical Physiology*, Summer 1959, Vol. 1, No. 1.

44. The Relative Influence of the Activity of Artificial and Breast Feeding on Facial Development. *Clinical Physiology*, Winter 1959, Vol. 1, No. 3.

45. Incidence of Poisoning from DDT and Other Chlorinated Hydrocarbon Insecticides. *Journal of Applied Nutrition*, Vol. 14, Nos. 2 & 3, pp. 140–145. (With Bernard Krohn, M.D.)

46. Poisoning from DDT and Other Chlorinated Hydrocarbon Pesticides: Pathogenesis, Diagnosis and Treatment. *Journal of Applied Nutrition*, Vol. 14, Nos. 2 & 3, pp. 126–138. (With Bernard Krohn, M.D.)

47. Reciprocal Relationship of Soil, Plant and Animal. *Missouri Agricultural Experiment Station Research Bulletin 765*.

48. A Fresh Look at Milk. *Clinical Physiology*, Winter 1961, Vol. 3, No. 3.

49. Milk—The Importance of Its Source. *Modern Nutrition*, Nov. 1961.

50. Nonspecific Methods for the Treatment of Allergic States. Discussion of presentations by L. P. Gay, Robert T. Pottenger, and G. F. Knight at the First Annual Convention of ICAN, Huntington-Sheraton, Pasadena, California. April 1961. Reprinted from the *Journal of Applied Nutrition*, Dec. 1964, Vol. 7, No. 4.

51. Which Are Boys and Which Are Girls? Weston A. Price Foundation, Inc. Santa Monica, California.

52. Applied Nutrition—President's Address. *Journal of Applied Nutrition*, 1965, Vol. 18, Nos. 1, 2, 3, & 4.

53. Does Social Practice Alter Man's Nutrition? (Editorial) *Journal of Applied Nutrition*, 1965, Vol. 18, Nos. 1, 2, 3, & 4.

54. What Can a County Medical Association Do about Air Pollution? *Archives of Environmental Health*, July 1967, Vol. 15.

55. Metabolic Factors of Development as Related to Physical Fitness. (Draft)

PRICE ℔ POTTENGER

Changing lives through **health and nutrition**

Until the publishing of this book, the experimental findings of The Cat Study were available only through Dr. Pottenger's published articles and a motion picture using his original films, now available on DVD (at www.price-pottenger.org). Compiled into one source, Dr. Pottenger's pioneering work is acquainting a vast, new audience with the importance of an adequate diet to health and longevity.

The Cat Study and its clinical applications join **Dr. Weston A. Price's** definitive volume, *Nutrition and Physical Degeneration*, as a classic in the field of nutrition. The message in these two books is as important today as when first published.

Where Dr. Pottenger's study of 900 cats shows that diets consisting of heat-processed milk and meat produced deficiency diseases and degenerative skeletal changes, Dr. Price's study of 14 primitive peoples shows that the introduction of processed, refined foods into their diets brought similar degenerative changes and increased susceptibility to infection.

We now know that the effect of small amounts of heat on food destroys enzymes and vitamins and alters the absorption and utilization of minerals. Both doctors' research tells us that unprocessed, natural foods are essential for the proper growth and development of the young and to the maintenance of good health.

Many people have at long last become interested in nutrition and are looking for guidance on how to incorporate nutrient-dense foods into their diets in order to attain exceptional health for themselves and future generations. Price-Pottenger is a nonprofit nutrition education foundation that offers online video courses, articles, tips, and live classes on nutrition and a wide variety of other topics that promote a healthier lifestyle. For decades, professionals have also turned to Price-Pottenger and its vast resources for information to improve the health of their clients.

Visit our website at www.price-pottenger.org, or contact us at our San Diego office: 7890 Broadway, Lemon Grove, CA 91945; (800) 366-3748 (U.S. only) or (619) 462-7600, Email: info@price-pottenger.org.

The Pottenger Cat Studies DVD

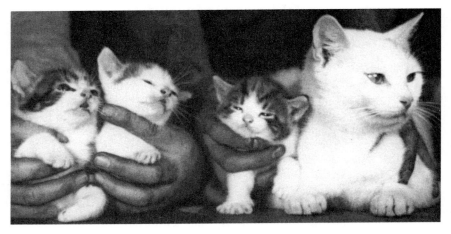

Raw Food Cat and Kittens
Photo copyright © Price-Pottenger, all rights reserved

This is a video of the famous 10-year nutrition study conducted by Francis M. Pottenger, Jr., MD, on more than 900 cats. The research documents how a diet of cooked meat and pasteurized milk led to progressive degeneration of the animals.

Comparison of healthy cats fed raw foods with those on heated foods is made, with mention of parallel findings among humans in Dr. Weston A. Price's worldwide studies. Behavioral characteristics, arthritis, sterility, skeletal deformities, and allergies are some of the problems the cats experienced that were associated with the consumption of a diet consisting entirely of cooked foods.

DVD 28.30 minutes
$30.00
$27.00 Member Price
Wholesale Discounts Available
Available at **www.price-pottenger.org**

ALL PRICES SUBJECT TO CHANGE WITHOUT NOTICE

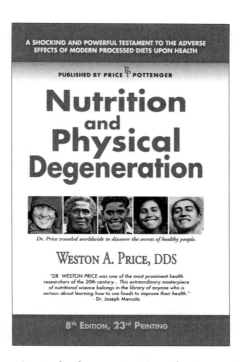

**An epic study demonstrating the importance
of whole food nutrition and the degeneration and
disease that comes from a diet of processed foods.**

For nearly 10 years, Weston Price and his wife traveled around the world in search of the secret
to health. Instead of looking at people afflicted with disease symptoms, this highly respected
dentist and researcher chose to focus on healthy individuals, and challenged himself to understand how they achieved such amazing health. Dr. Price traveled to hundreds of cities in a total
of 14 countries in his search to find healthy people. He investigated some of the most remote
areas in the world and observed perfect dental arches, minimal tooth decay, high immunity to
tuberculosis, and overall excellent health in those groups of people who ate their indigenous
foods. He found when these people were introduced to modernized foods, such as white flour,
white sugar, refined vegetable oils, and canned goods, signs of degeneration quickly became
evident. Dental caries, deformed jaw structures, crooked teeth, arthritis, and a low immunity
to tuberculosis became rampant among them. Dr. Price documented this ancestral wisdom—
including hundreds of photos—in his book, *Nutrition and Physical Degeneration.*

WESTON A. PRICE – *"Life in all its fullness is mother nature obeyed."*

Weston A. Price, DDS
Includes 196 photos and 6 maps
527 pages, softcover
$27.95
$25.15 Member Price
Wholesale Discounts Available

Available at **www.price–pottenger.org**

Dr. Price's Search for Health DVD

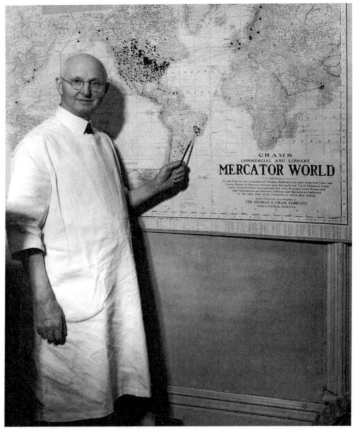

This is an overview of the research of Dr. Weston A. Price, DDS, revealing the effect of diet on native peoples around the world. It vividly shows that dental caries, misalignment of teeth, increased susceptibility to disease, and physical and mental degeneration are largely attributed to the use of modern processed foods, and that optimal health starts with sound nutrition from whole foods from both vegetable and animal sources, eaten fresh or prepared with methods that do not remove essential fats, vitamins, and minerals.

DVD 25.30 minutes
$35.00
$31.50 Member Price
Wholesale Discounts Available
Available at **www.price-pottenger.org**

ALL PRICES SUBJECT TO CHANGE WITHOUT NOTICE

Dental Infections, Oral and Systemic & Dental Infections and The Degenerative Diseases, Vol 1 & 2

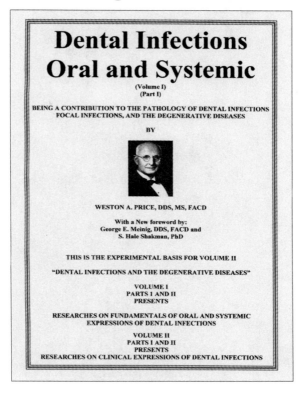

Weston A. Price, DDS, conducted a 25-year project under the auspices of the American Dental Association's Research Institute, on the subject of infected teeth and how they cause disease. This is Dr. Price's complete research report:

Volume 1: A contribution to the pathology of dental infections, focal infections, and the degenerative diseases (experimental basis).

Includes 262 illustrations with 8 color illustrations and 261 charts

Volume 2: Researches on clinical expressions of dental infections.

Includes 6 color illustrations

Weston A. Price, DDS
1174 pages, 2 volumes in four parts, steel spine bound by Price-Pottenger
$150.00
$135.00 Member Price
Available at **www.price-pottenger.org**

ALL PRICES SUBJECT TO CHANGE WITHOUT NOTICE

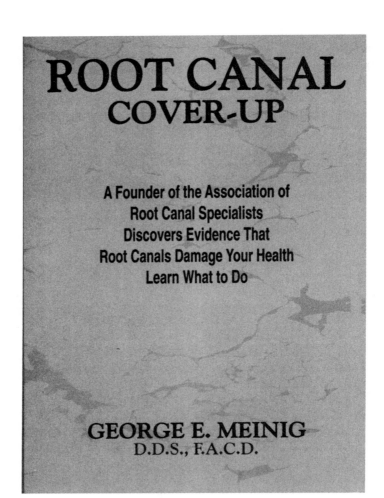

ROOT CANAL
COVER-UP

**A Founder of the Association of
Root Canal Specialists
Discovers Evidence That
Root Canals Damage Your Health
Learn What to Do**

GEORGE E. MEINIG
D.D.S., F.A.C.D.

Root Canal Cover-Up shows how hidden bacteria in teeth cause side effects that can endanger your life. Discover how germs trapped in teeth and tonsils mutate and metastasize like cancer cells and how these bacteria migrate to heart, kidney, eye, brain, arthritic joints, and countless other parts of the body. Learn how Dr. Meinig discovered that a meticulous 25-year research project conducted by Weston A. Price, DDS, under the auspices of the American Dental Association's Research Institute, was buried by disbelievers of the focal infection theory.

George E. Meinig, DDS, FACD
227 pages, softcover
$19.95
$17.95 Member Price
Wholesale Discounts Available
Available at **www.price-pottenger.org**

ALL PRICES SUBJECT TO CHANGE WITHOUT NOTICE

The Price-Pottenger Story DVD

Morley Video Productions, Licensed to Price-Pottenger

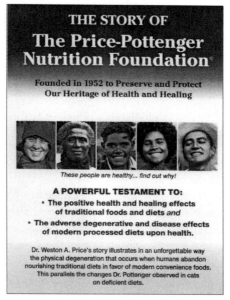

The story of Price-Pottenger, as well as that of Drs. Price and Pottenger's research, is now available on one DVD. In three parts, Janet and Don Morley have created a wonderful gift to Price-Pottenger by presenting this valuable information.

Part 1 – The Price/Pottenger Studies

This section is a synopsis of the works of Dr. Weston A. Price, DDS, and Dr. Francis M. Pottenger, Jr., MD. The stories of Dr. Price's and Dr. Pottenger's studies are intermixed with modern relevance, which shows that the findings from their research of many years ago are still relevant today.

Part 2 – The Foundation: The Story of Price-Pottenger

The history of the foundation told through staff interviews from our beginning to where we are today and where we are going in the future.

Part 3 – Staff Interviews

The complete interviews that are partially used throughout the entire DVD.

DVD 1 hour and 25 minutes
$25.00
$20.00 Member Price
Wholesale Discounts Available
Available at **www.price-pottenger.org**

ALL PRICES SUBJECT TO CHANGE WITHOUT NOTICE

Become a Member

Join Price-Pottenger, an educational nonprofit committed to keeping you healthy. Prevent cancer, heart disease, diabetes, and the other degenerative conditions that threaten your well-being.

Visit **price-pottenger.org** to access the many exclusive benefits available to our members and health professionals. Sign up for a *free one-month trial membership* and explore topics such as Nutrition, Recipes and Food Preparation, Natural Medicine, Vitamins and Minerals, Dental Health, Fertility and Prenatal Nutrition, Antiaging, Detoxification, Mental Health, and more.

Become part of the community that has discovered the power of traditional foods and the rewards that come from a truly healthy lifestyle. Reclaim your health and join the organization that, for over 60 years, has been helping people feel better, live better, and live longer. *Sign up today!*

**www.price-pottenger.org • info@price-pottenger.org •
1-800-366-3748 (U.S. only) • 619-462-7600**

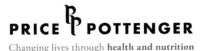

PRICE ℔ POTTENGER

Changing lives through **health and nutrition**

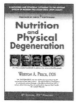 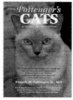 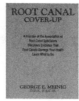